INTERFACE

MECHANISMS OF SPIRIT
IN OSTEOPATHY

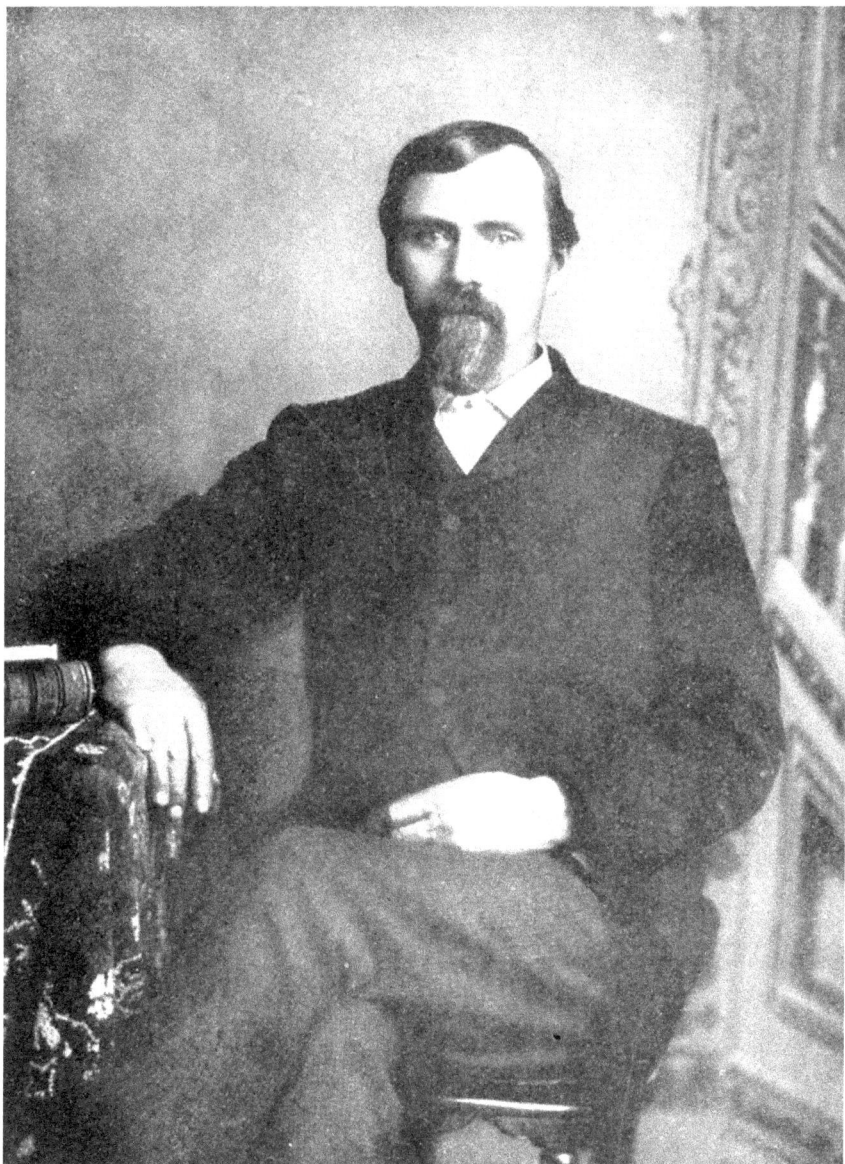

Photograph of A. T. Still seated at a desk.
(Reproduced from the inside cover of the original 1897 edition of *Autobiography of A. T. Still*.)

INTERFACE

Mechanisms of Spirit
in Osteopathy

R. PAUL LEE, DO

Published by:
Stillness Press, LLC
www.stillnesspress.com

Fifth Printing 2023

Cover and book design by Lubosh Cech *luboshcech.com*

Grateful acknowledgement is made to the Sutherland Cranial Teaching Foundation for permission to use quotations of William G. Sutherland that appear in *Teachings in the Science of Osteopathy* and *Contributions of Thought.*

ISBN 978-0-9675851-3-0 Hardcover
ISBN 979-8-9875675-1-7 Softcover
ISBN 979-8-9875675-2-4 eBook

Ordering information: Stillness Press, LLC books available at www.stillnesspress.com

This book is dedicated to Robert Fulford, DO,
who inducted me with Osteopathy's spirit.

Mind and Matter
In Reciprocity
The Yang and Yin
Of Osteopathy

Love of God
Which Underlies The All
The Breath of Life
Creates Life from What's Still

Life is Motion
Said Andrew Taylor Still
An Interface
To Physicality

ACKNOWLEDGMENTS

I wish to acknowledge the many influential people in my life who have led me to the writing of this book. I especially thank the wisdom and great care that Rachel Brooks provided in advising me about the contents and style of this book. She is a wonderful editor. I took her sincere suggestions as the best choice, except one. I give a special thanks of appreciation to Tony Chila, who has supported my growth in the osteopathic realm as teacher, advisor, and writer of the foreword to this book. Lawrence Bellew and other interested osteopathic physicians provided me along the way with important articles from the scientific literature. My parents directed me to be diligent and thorough. Perhaps I am now accomplishing what it was that they always imagined for me. I regret that they are no longer alive to join me in celebrating, but I acknowledge their ongoing awareness and support. There are so many teachers and authors who shaped my thinking. I would like to name a few: Patricia Spradling, Fritjof Capra, Larry Dossey, Carlos Castaneda, Brugh Joy, Barbara Ann Brennan, Ted J. Kaptchuk, Kenneth R. Pelletier, Richard Gerber, Björn E.W. Nordenström, Alfred Pischinger. More recently, I have been influenced by other great scientists and thinkers including David Bohm, William Tiller, and Joseph Rael.

From within my profession of osteopathic medicine, those who influenced my thinking, in the order in which they came into my life, include Andrew Taylor Still; Fred L. Mitchell, Jr.; Kendall Hall; William W. Lemley; William Garner Sutherland; Paula L. Eschtruth; Robert C. Fulford; J. Scott Heatherington; Lawrence Jones; Paul E. Kimberly; Viola M. Frymann; Edna M. Lay; Rollin E. Becker; Herbert C. Miller; Anthony G. Chila; James S. Jealous; Larry W. Bader; William A. Kuchera; Michael L. Kuchera; Michael D. Lockwood; Harold D. Goodman; John H. Harakal; Irvin M. Korr; Anne L. Wales; Jean-Pierre Barral; Bernard Gabarel; Michel Roques; John Adams; Carlisle Holland; Alan R. Becker; Bonnie R. Gintis; Hugh M. Ettlinger; Harold I. Magoun, Jr.; Rachel E. Brooks; Louis Hasbrouck; Paul E. Dart; Margaret A. Sorrel; Charlotte Weaver; Kenneth J. Lossing; and Zachary Comeaux. There are also others, who remain unnamed but who influenced these. Mostly, I thank my patients for the ultimate teaching, and I thank Creator for gifting me with who I am as a human being and what I am as an osteopathic physician, able to do this work that I love so well.

CONTENTS

FOREWORD

The 21st century has arrived and is now moving forward in its appointed course in time. While it may seem to some that the original thought process of Andrew Taylor Still is dated (19th century), the advances in knowledge of the 20th century have provided more challenges to explain this visionary's contribution to the practice of medicine. This is the daunting task undertaken by the author, R. Paul Lee, DO.

Andrew Taylor Still often described his contribution as a Philosophy, Science, and Art. A comparison of paradigms of thought before and after Still shows a significant overlap in the categorizations of Energy, Matter, and Life Form. It is in regard to the latter that early osteopathic students, teachers, and authors have expended great effort to grasp and continue the advancement of Still's original thought. It is on this point that one can better appreciate the significance of the work of William G. Sutherland.

In this book, a model is proposed that attempts to explain the accomplishment of physical phenomena through the primary respiratory mechanism. In its development, this model reviews and offers a further analysis of Still's teaching. In addition, the elaborating work of Still's student, William G. Sutherland, is given a reappraisal in the light of contemporary cellular physiology.

An exhaustive analysis of studies that have a bearing on the connective tissue system of the body helps our appreciation of the complexity of Still's thought. In the process of synthesizing sources, the emergence of key considerations devolves to the behavior of water as a unit, the material importance of the connective tissue, and the interface of form and motion.

Motion is perceived as the special characteristic that produces Health. Water and electricity are the media that relate the dichotomy of the life-form's energetic and physical realms. Osteopathic Manipulative Treatment is the means for addressing structural distortion, allowing the return of Health. Modalities of treatment aside, Health must be restored from within. The Tide then delivers Health.

The Tide is evaluated in its biochemical characteristics. In a detailed, practical, and theoretical process, the author considers the entirety of contemporary cellular physiology. It is an outcome of this process that leads the practitioner to the necessity of recognizing the holistic value of working with a holographic system. The summation of this recognition comes with the achievement of the stillness of oscillation, the transmuting effect of the exchange between all fluid compartments of the organism. It is in the moment of exchange that metabolic power is reset.

The reader who is familiar with osteopathic theory and practice will appreciate the effort to bring a better level of scientific understanding to bear on the cognitive and experiential aspects of both. The reader not familiar with osteopathic theory and practice will perhaps be challenged to explore broader horizons of meaning in the practice of medicine. In reading this book, each will be asked to confront information with personal knowledge.

Anthony G. Chila, DO, FAAO

Professor, Department of Family Medicine
Ohio University College of Osteopathic Medicine

INTRODUCTION

Students come to osteopathic medicine for many and varied reasons. Some come because a grandparent or parent was a Doctor of Osteopathy (DO). Others come to find an alternative means to practice allopathic medicine. Yet others feel the desire to offer to people what is uniquely Osteopathy's to offer. I came to this profession because I wanted to practice medicine but I was not admitted to allopathic medical school. Yet I recognized as I visited physicians as a pharmaceutical representative that most of the doctors on my call list with DO after their names had a different attitude than most of those with MD.

So, when some of the osteopathic physicians in my territory offered to assist me with my application to the Kansas City College of Osteopathic Medicine, I felt that my prayer to be a doctor had been answered. It was answered in a special way because I saw the opportunity to be one of those doctors who openly cared for patients and collaborated with them for their improved health. Although I didn't know what a DO was, I knew I would eventually find out. Well, I have been surprised to discover how long it has taken me to understand and that my understanding continues to grow, even to the time of this writing.

I entered osteopathic medical school with tremendous desire and succeeded as a student because of it; but, at graduation, I still did not know what a DO was. At that time in the history of the Kansas City College of Osteopathic Medicine, by a quirk of fate, there was a gap in the teaching of Osteopathic Principles and Practice (OPP). The administration could not find OPP faculty for one year of my basic science education, and my query, "What is a DO?" remained largely unanswered. I knew that I needed to crack a neck or back if there was a restriction of motion responsible for symptoms. I even knew that I could do it—usually—without hurting the subject of my violence. As for anything else related to OPP, I did not comprehend why the technique was to be applied except to relieve pain. I did not realize where the idea of Osteopathy originated from. I could not understand why there were two separate but equal medical professions. My subsequent training in the clinical years and internship offered me no further osteopathic insights.

Entering practice, I was confronted with many patients who complained of back, neck, or head pain or of dysfunctions of the extremities or viscera. I recognized that I needed to learn more about this black hole of "find it, fix it, and leave it alone." I wanted to be able to palpate what was wrong and to correct it. I wanted to understand the mechanisms of dysfunction. Then, J. Scott Heatherington, DO, introduced me to strain-counterstrain, an osteopathic manipulative technique that appeared magical to me. I sputtered, how can motion be regained and pain relieved by holding a body part in one place for 90 seconds? Fascination with this modality took me a long way for many years, until I found cranial osteopathy. As it says on the chamber of commerce brochure in spectacular mountainous Chaffee County, Colorado: "Now THIS is Colorado!" I knew I had found Osteopathy when I found the cranial concept. I said to myself, now THIS is Osteopathy! I have come to the mountain!

But I still did not understand. I asked myself, what is making this tide that I can palpate? How can I palpate inside the body when my hands are on the surface? What is going on biochemically? Biochemistry had been my "religion" in undergraduate school, where I majored in comparative biochemistry and physiology. It proved for me the existence of God, a universal plan, iterations of function that I could identify at all levels from biochemistry to astronomy. In that era, Watson and Crick had just elucidated the structure of DNA, and the ribosomes had just been discovered as microscopic conveyor belts in a protein-assembly plant. On the level of cellular physiology, these are mechanisms of life. They represent the life force just as much as animated speech, graceful dance, or brilliant thought express life, relative to the whole individual.

The next series of questions that came to my mind were: How does thought manifest as speech, movement, or another thought? For that matter, does thought create healing? If manipulation creates healing, how does it work? Is there an answer in biochemistry? What is a still point? How does it effect a transmutation? What is transmutation? And, Oh! by the way, what is Osteopathy?

All these questions made me look to the source of it all, Andrew Taylor Still, MD, DO. At the suggestion of Dr. Heatherington, I decided to go to Kirksville for a residency in Osteopathic Manipulative Medicine. There, I encountered the essence of Dr. Still. Today, I continue to dig into his mind to reach a greater understanding. What a wealth of information. What an insightful man. What a concurrence of thought with so many other great thinkers, both ancient and modern. What a pity the profession he founded does not embrace the essence of his thought. But many people did not embrace his philosophy when he was alive either. Osteopathy has always been ahead of its time—until now. Now, greater and greater numbers of people are eager to hear the message from Drew Still.

The mind-set of western culture is prepared, even hungry, for a re-connection with spirit that it has denied for centuries. Until now, science has provided mechanical answers to heart-felt questions. But modern physics now demonstrates that mysticism and mathematics mingle. Both disciplines produce similar solutions. Non-locality, a principle of modern physics, explains many heretofore unexplainable phenomena relative to spirit: the power of prayer, psychokinesis, and precognition, to name a few. There is a practicality to spirit when one examines it objectively. Spirit is real, a substance, palpable. The tide is a manifestation of spirit. We can work directly with spirit—with our hands. It's very pragmatic. For me, it begins to take the mystery out of what I grew up knowing about spirit in the context of religion.

Dr. Still understood that spirit continues after death. He held séances with his neighbors, Spiritualists and Swedenborgians, who founded Lawrence, Kansas, in the 1850s. They arrived by Conestoga wagons from Massachusetts to assure that Kansas would be a free state, not a slave state. These open-minded and searching people offered Drew Still the like-mindedness that he needed to develop his philosophy. Still was convinced of the perfection of creation—of the perfection of the structure and function of the human body. He knew he could work with its structure to improve its function. He was convinced that his ideas were based on essential truths found in nature, where he derived his inspiration.

Today there is a ground swell of interest in such topics—integrating spirit with other aspects of life. Osteopathy can provide a context for such integration. Still's Osteopathy is spirit in action. Healing occurs because spirit provides the impetus. One can feel it occur under one's hands when one feels the primary respiratory mechanism. It struggles to free the tissue that cannot receive health; it brings that tissue into synchrony with the remainder; then it becomes still; and finally it resumes an "easy normal" or healthy fluctuation. This is how healing happens. The action of healing is palpable.

Healing happens with or without a medical diagnosis. If there is a structural component to a disease process, and there inevitably is, it can be treated with osteopathic manipulative treatment (OMT). OMT may or may not cure the disease process, but it will, at least, improve the level of functioning of the organism enough to bring it into a new balance with the disturbance of function that is associated with the disease process. This new balance might ameliorate or completely dissipate the symptoms and signs of disease.

With OMT, we are dealing with the forces of healing, not the naming of disease. That is not to say that the name of the disease is unimportant or that the mechanisms of pathology should be denied. And, furthermore, that is not to say that the exact structural diagnosis of somatic dysfunction has no value.

Dr. Still advised us to visualize the normal anatomy to promote healing. OMT brings in the health according to the ability of the operator to visualize how the disturbance in the tissues looks in health. If we know what is wrong—what is the pathology—then we have a place to begin. But we do not treat what is wrong. We treat by assisting the patient's body to reestablish the original perfection with which each of us entered the material world. The manner in which we assist the body to re-order the distortion to return to the perfection of the original is by visualizing the original. Our images become critical to our success. Our nervous systems reflect these images and the patient receives them through our hands and our minds. The morphogenetic field is there as a reference, the water is the mediator, and the piezoelectric connective tissue is ready to receive. These concepts are addressed in detail in this book.

William Harvey's great contribution to science[1] in the 1600s was that the flow of blood within the vessels of the body describes a one-way continuous circulation, as opposed to the popular notion of his day that blood nourished the tissues through an ebb-and-flow motion. William G. Sutherland's great contribution to science in the 1900s was that the metabolic activity resulting from this continuous one-way delivery of nutrients describes an ebb-and-flow fluctuation in the interstitium and cells rather than today's popular notion that diffusion alone distributes nutrients.[2]

A respiratory fluctuation, Sutherland proclaimed, orders the metabolic activity of nutrient delivery and waste disposal. There is an organized process, not mere chance, that determines the biochemical activities of the cell and its environment. The connective tissues are the tissues that do the organizing. With water as the mediator, the fibrous elements of the cell and the interstitium provide the means by which the system operates biomechanically, biochemically, and bioelectrically. Even the lymphatic channels synchronize with this oscillatory behavior of the tissue matrix system.

Sutherland referred to the Bible and to Dr. Still to declare that spirit is responsible for this respiratory rhythm—an independent, palpable oscillation. These palpable activities are mechanisms of spirit. All the tissues participate. It is fundamental to life. Someday Sutherland's discovery may receive the recognition it deserves, along with Harvey's, as one of physiology's all-time greatest discoveries.

Sutherland's contention that an ebb-and-flow phenomenon underlies metabolism came not only from information obtained from an extrapolation of Still's ideas and texts but also from knowledge obtained from research and clinical experience, originally demonstrated on his own head and eventually through his patients and students. Such knowledge supersedes any need for a scientific proof of the existence of the phenomenon because it is in and of itself *prima facie* evidence of its existence. Beyond a basic observation by palpation, scientific proof is merely a tool needed to demonstrate how, when, and why it happens, not whether it does. Science demonstrates to those who do not observe a particular phenomenon firsthand by some objective measurement that the phenomenon is real. But scientific proof is not necessary for those who directly observe the phenomenon.

My desire to understand osteopathic philosophy and practice led me on a long and varied expedition. At first, my biochemical orientation forged a desire in me to diagnose illness in the manner of an allopathic internist. But I recognized that the disease model of medicine alone would limit my ability to expand my view beyond the physical manifestations of illness. It was clear to me that most illness generates from emotional and mental sources that demand of the physician a wide perspective of the human condition that a purely physical assessment cannot fully address.

Through the process of discovery, I became an advocate for Osteopathy. As a reformed smoker advocates for clean air, I moved from categorizing patients by their diseases to observing their bodies' potential for healing. I wondered what occurred under my hands that allowed me to feel when healing happens. In scientific terms, what mechanism in the tissues explains this palpable phenomenon? Why do injured tissues feel indurated, ropy, and resistant to movement? Why do these tissues immediately become supple and movable with osteopathic manipulative treatment? What is healing compared to curing disease?

While these questions about the physiological mechanisms in the tissues filled my head, another set of questions was swirling about with equal force. Since osteopathic medicine seems to offer such an advantage, why is it that so many patients could not routinely avail themselves of its healing? What forces keep so many who need OMT from receiving it? Why do pregnant mothers and newborns not routinely receive OMT? Why do those in chronic pain not have the wholesale opportunity to receive the benefits of OMT?

Whereas allopathic medicine has its greatest strength in making pathological diagnoses in acute medical and surgical conditions, osteopathic medicine provides a template for other approaches to long-term healing that can be integrated with acute care medicine. I discovered that allopathic medicine's successes, although great, needed the supplementary approach that osteopathic medicine brings to the bedside.

Osteopathic medicine's greatest contribution to the health of society comes not by looking at statistical averages and making a diagnosis fit a person but rather by looking at what the tissues of the individual patient report to the physician's palpatory diagnostic skill at that moment in time. Disturbances of health respond to careful examination and specific treatment of particular findings in an individual rather than offering up the individual to chance based on population percentages.

One of the great hallmarks of osteopathic medicine's success is the care expressed by the physician for his or her patient. This caring emanates directly from the individual attention the osteopathic physician must give to the patient in order to do his or her palpatory work. The DO finds the health in the individual's body and promotes its expression. This is the benefit that all patients should have available to them.

This book offers to proponents of osteopathic medicine philosophic considerations based on science and clinical experience to preserve the distinctiveness and viability of the profession. The rationale for this purpose appears in this book as: (1) a review of the medical and scientific literature, which supports (2) a new, expanded model of the osteopathic philosophy, which (3) reinterprets Still's philosophy and (4) reinvigorates the reason for the existence of the osteopathic medical profession. This book expresses my work to fulfill the meaning of "DO" as Dr. Still interpreted it for his first graduates: "Dig On."

In this book, I explore the philosophy of osteopathic medicine from the perspectives of its science and art. In Chapter One, I review in some detail the philosophy given to us by Andrew Taylor Still, MD, DO, and in Chapters Two and Three, I explore the supporting evidence for his philosophy by other thinkers and authors. Then, in Chapter Four, I present scientific evidence for a new model of the science, art, and philosophy of osteopathic medicine. Chapter Five summarizes the new model. In the Appendix, I list the basic assumptions of Still's philosophy, as I understand them, in today's terms. The profession can succeed by being proactive about what makes it unique. Leaving this to others will not spell success and denies patients a distinctive approach to healing that could relieve suffering that would otherwise not be alleviated.

My hope is that the reader will receive something beneficial from reading this book, both personally and professionally. I certainly have benefited from the exercise of writing it by gaining greater understanding about the way things work: osteopathically, physiologically, and spiritually.

1

THE MAN AND HIS PHILOSOPHY

Spirit put the stamp of individuality on Itself, and called it you.
—— ERNEST HOLMES

Andrew Taylor Still, MD, DO, crafted *de novo* a philosophy and practice of medicine unique and powerful enough to effect healings in many people who were otherwise unalleviated and to produce a distinctive medical profession that persists today despite more than a century of trials. Chapter One examines Dr. Still's philosophy and his practice of Osteopathy.* This chapter reviews those attributes of Still's philosophy that have earned the osteopathic medical profession its place in history and society: its uniqueness, power for healing, and worthiness as a force for change. First, this chapter discusses our modern interpretation of Still's philosophy. Then, it compares that interpretation with what Andrew Still, himself, said about his "child, Osteopathy." It also

---

* I capitalize "Osteopathy" in this book to cherish A. T. Still's vision with reverence and signify that Osteopathy is a spiritual reality.

explores evidence about Dr. Still's character and experience to help us understand his personal view of his world and his form of medicine.

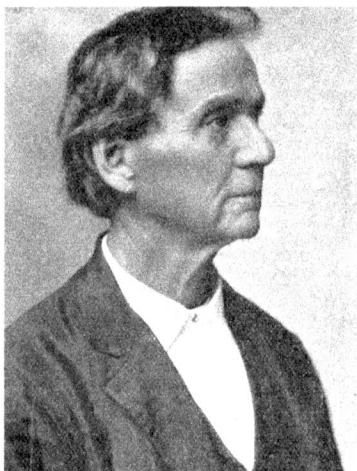

1.1 Photograph of Dr. A. T. Still without his beard, ca.1900. Courtesy of Still National Osteopathic Museum, Kirksville, MO.

This opening chapter, an intimate review of A. T. Still's ideas and where they came from, clearly points to *spirit* as the fundamental generative source of all that he declared and taught as his healing philosophy and practice, Osteopathy. Spirit, not religion, is the subject of this book and, starting with this chapter, we dissect the ideas relative to spirit as Still propounded them. The word "spirit" holds many different connotations for different people, and some may want to reject the notion that the original philosophy was based on spirit. This only serves to limit Still's legacy. As this book will show, spirit in Osteopathy turns out to be scientific, practical, and very useful in a medical model that osteopathic physicians can readily abide.

Dr. Still wanted us to embellish his bold strokes of basic truths. He said that although he had discovered a new creature, he had only "grasped the tail of the squirrel in the hole of the tree."[1] He expected us, who have inherited his revelation, to deliver the "critter" and submit it to detailed examination, interpretation, elucidation, and exposition. Drew Still believed that he had revealed a fundamental truth of nature and asserted that we must explore it and expand our understanding of it as new information is discovered. By doing so, we will comprehend all the better the essence of nature, improve our effectiveness in working with her healing potential, and increase our personal, professional, and universal benefits from such knowledge and skill.

I. OSTEOPATHY'S MODERN DEFINITION AND STILL'S DEFINITION

A. Modern Definition

The modern interpretation of Still's philosophy, quoting from the present publications of the osteopathic medical profession, is as follows:

> Osteopathic medicine is a philosophy of health care and a distinctive art, supported by expanding scientific knowledge; its philosophy embraces the concept of the unity of the living organism's structure (anatomy) and function (physiology). Its art is the application of the philosophy in the practice of medicine and surgery and all its branches and specialties. Its science includes the behavioral, chemical, physical, spiritual and biological knowledge related to the establishment and maintenance of health as well as the prevention and alleviation of disease. Osteopathic concepts emphasize the following principles: 1) The human being is a dynamic unit of function; 2) The body possesses self-regulatory mechanisms, which are self-healing in nature; 3) Structure and function are interrelated at all levels; 4) Rational treatment is based on these principles.[2]

Although correct as far as it goes, this official definition from the osteopathic profession is admittedly abbreviated. These brief words attempt to summarize four volumes of Still's writings,[3–6] many volumes that have been written about Still and his philosophy by other authors (some of which are referenced here),[7–13] and a century of research and clinical experience by a growing profession that presently numbers nearly 50,000 fully licensed physicians in the United States representing multiple specialties and many Osteopaths around the world with privileges according to their countries' regulations. All of this literature, research, and clinical experience obviously challenges any brief summary of the osteopathic philosophy to be fully representative and inclusive. More to the point, this official definition lacks essential elements of the osteopathic philosophy as Still enunciated it. In his writings, Still propounded, as part of his philosophy, fundamental principles that today the profession largely excludes from its definition. We will examine the timing and possible reasons for this omission.

In February 2002, a multidisciplinary ad hoc committee appointed by the American Osteopathic Association (AOA) announced its "proposed tenets of osteopathic medicine" and "principles for patient care."[14] The AOA offered these tenets and principles as a starting point for comment and discussion within the osteopathic medical profession, the goal of which was to create philosophical guidelines that would stand the test of time and invite individual interpretation. The tenets were stated as follows:

1. A person is the product of dynamic interaction between body, mind, and spirit.

2. An inherent property of this dynamic interaction is the capacity of the individual for the maintenance of health and the recovery from disease.

3. Many forces, both intrinsic and extrinsic to the person, can challenge this inherent capacity and contribute to the onset of illness.

4. The musculoskeletal system significantly influences the individual's ability to restore this inherent capacity and therefore to resist disease processes.

The stated principles for patient care were (1) the patient is the focus for health care, (2) the patient has the primary responsibility for his or her health, and (3) an effective treatment program for patient care is founded on these tenets.

It is heartening that the AOA is working to redefine the stated purpose for the existence of the osteopathic medical profession. Nevertheless, this most recent version continues to exclude important concepts from A. T. Still. It is critical to include these forgotten ideas if we are to capture the core of Still's concepts and to express the essence of the effectiveness of his methods. This book contributes to this discussion of the tenets and the principles for patient care within the ongoing osteopathic profession.

If we were to entertain and then to find ways to implement the forgotten but essential spiritual elements of Andrew Still's philosophy, it would change the course of the profession's progress and development. These unmentioned principles could help solve the identity crisis that has encumbered the osteopathic medical profession. They could also provide a distinct advantage to the profession in its evolution within the current medical milieu, in which both conventional and unconventional methods are fomenting a new breed of practitioner. The osteopathic medical profession could take a leadership role in this mix by demonstrating how to integrate orthodox and unorthodox practices. In the process, osteopathic medicine might rediscover itself and integrate its precepts more thoroughly into every aspect of its broad reach. If the profession were to adopt these powerful precepts given to us from Still, the revolution that he envisioned could potently proceed, and all of medicine might apprehend a new horizon.

(1) **Timidity takes possession of us only when we are at a loss to judge of the end from the beginning.** (Still, in Booth, 42)

As we see when we examine his philosophy, Still tapped into ideas that today, after more than 100 years, many people consider to be innovative and worthy of adoption. Osteopathy will become the leader in this innovation in medicine that is presently underway if the profession fully acknowledges its roots. To do so, we must fully comprehend what he said and what he meant.

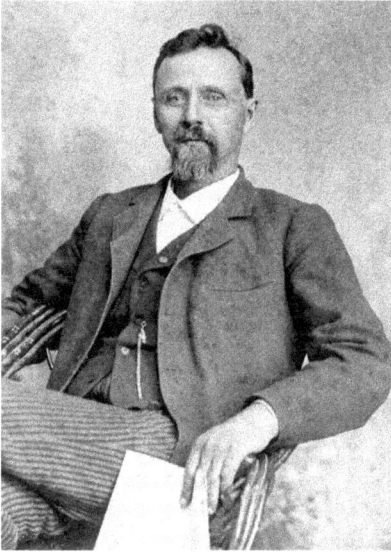

1.2 Dr. A. T. Still in wicker chair with newspaper, 1895. Courtesy Still National Osteopathic Museum, Kirksville, MO.

B. Still's Simplified Definition

Charlotte Weaver, DO, was a student of A. T. Still who took up his challenge to research how osteopathic principles relate to the human cranium and dedicated her life to it. She indicated that on several occasions Dr. Still verbally provided her with this simplified definition of Osteopathy:

(2) Normal structure in normal juxtaposition means normal function.
With especial stress upon the osseous tissues.[15]

Of course, Still had much more to say about his philosophy than this short statement. We will look at his writings in detail, but first let us look at where his ideas came from.

C. Genesis of Osteopathy

Great spirits always encounter violent opposition by mediocre minds.
— ALBERT EINSTEIN

1. Rational and Scientific Medicine

Still's ideas were generated, in part, from the same desire that subsequently changed all of medicine after the Flexner Report in 1911, that is, to place the practice of medicine on a more scientific basis. Article III of the Constitution (1894) for the American School of Osteopathy states:

> (3) The object of this corporation is to establish a College of Osteopathy, the design of which is to improve our present system of surgery, obstetrics, and treatment of diseases generally, and place the same on a more *rational and scientific* basis, and to impart information to the medical profession. . . . (Still 1908, 142; italics added)

He was appalled by the use of the poisonous, ineffective, or addictive remedies of the day, which he also used. He felt that medical doctors poorly understood normal human function and disease and comprehended even less well the kinds of drugs, their effects, and uses.

2. Beginnings

Dr. Still indicated that Osteopathy is derived from Divine principles of nature, merely waiting to be discovered:

> (4) We take up Osteopathy. How old is it? Give me the age of God

and I will give you the age of Osteopathy. It is a law of mind, matter, and motion. (Still 1908, 29)

(5) Age after age has passed, and if this science was ever known, the historians have failed to record any part of it for the use of their successors. I feel it is a debt I owe to the nineteenth century, to at least begin to fill the blank with the truths of Osteopathy which have been before all centuries of the past, asking: "And shall I travel the lonely road of another century and not be noticed by man?" (Still 1908, 151)

In 1855,* when Andrew Still, his family, and their neighbors were driven from their homes in the Kansas Territory during a raid from pro-slavery forces from Missouri, Major James Burnett Abbott, "a close, personal, and intimate friend" of Still, said to him while they were hiding in the woods, "Do you know that I have lost all faith in medicine? I am satisfied that it is all wrong, and that the system of drugs, as curative agents, will some day be practically overturned, and some other system or method of curing the sick without drugs will take its place in healing the sick" (Abbott, in Booth, 45). Col. A. L. Conger reported, "Major Abbott was formerly from the state of Connecticut; a man who was thoroughly scientific and had great learning. The words of Major Abbott made a deep and lasting impression on the mind of Dr. Still, and the more he thought of the suggestion, the more it seemed to him that he was to be the instrument through which this overthrowing of drugs was to be brought about, and some other and better system was to be given to mankind" (Conger, in Booth, 46).

Once this seed was planted, Still's ideas came to him—a gifted, eccentric, and intuitive genius (Booth, 13–43)—from his observation

------

* Booth stated that Still met Abbott in 1858; however, the skirmishes related to the slavery issue in eastern Kansas mostly ended in 1857, making Trowbridge's date of 1855 more plausible. See Trowbridge C (1991). Andrew Taylor Still: 1828–1917. Kirksville, MO: Thomas Jefferson University Press, 57, 63.

of nature, study of anatomy, and reflection on creation. His keen ability to observe the whole of reality, coupled with raw inspiration and galvanized by personal hardship, propelled his thinking to break out of the standard mold and to attempt to satisfy his hunger for knowledge about nature, life, and humans. This search resulted in his discovery and development of a new system of medicine that pragmatically applies ancient themes and principles of nature to human health (Still 1908; Booth).

For Still's philosophy of medicine to emerge from within him, he had to step outside the customary mind-set of the medical practitioners of his day. By comparing his singularity against the masses of authors recommending the drugs of his day, he acknowledged his unique approach:

> (6) I will not worry your patience with a list of the names of authors that have written upon the subject of drugs as remedial agents. I will use the word that the theologian often uses when asked for whom Christ died: the answer universally is, All." (Still 1892, 10)

Knowing that his ideas opposed those of the vast majority, Still referred to his process by comparing himself to others who left the mainstream:

> (7) The masses are not Galileos, Washingtons, nor Lincolns, but now and then a Fulton, a Clay, a Grant, an Edison arises, or some unchained mind moves against tradition, with an unerring philosophy. (Still 1908, 226)

He realized that his new science, Osteopathy, would not blend with the mainstream and that its acceptance could not be guaranteed. He indicated in 1895 that the place on which it stood was

(8) defiant, offensive, and defensive, for Osteopathy has had to take each position. It could not come to the place due it and offend no one. Old and established theories and professions claim the right to say who shall live or die, and have claimed this prerogative so long that they feel offended at the birth of any new child of progress that comes upon the stage to ask a hearing without their permission. Then to defend would be inseparable from the growth of the science, as merit is above all tribunals except God Himself. (Still 1908, 163)

In reference to the acceptance of Osteopathy, Dr. Still related in his autobiography, a story about his Kirksville friend, Mr. Harris, who said, "Dr. Still, in my opinion a man dreads that which he does not comprehend" (Still 1908, 227). Still commented:

(9) That was his answer twenty-two years ago, and that is the reason osteopathy is not accepted by the masses and is not adopted by every man and woman of intelligence to-day. A man dreads to give up his old boots for fear the new ones will pinch his feet. We have gone from generation to generation imitating the habits of our ancestors. (Still 1908, 227)

As Booth comments, "It has been said that the trouble with most men is not that they know too much, but that they know so much that is not true. When we think of the abandoned theories and the discarded practices of the medical profession, we conclude that that saying applies especially to those whose very title, doctor, designates them as learned. What Dr. Still learned from nature was true and did not have to be unlearned. Whenever he got the scent of truth he followed the trail wherever it led. If to error, he abandoned it; if to truth, he laid firm hold upon it" (Booth, 49). "He believed that osteopathy is synonymous with truth, and it would gradually unfold and develop into perfect symmetry. That is what gave him the courage to carry on his work under the most adverse and trying conditions" (Booth, 63–64). And as W. G. Sutherland said in 1950, "In seventy-five years in the crucible of time, not one statement made by Dr. A. T. Still has needed revising.[16]

In his autobiography, Still commented about his explorations that led to his new philosophy:

> (10) My science or discovery was born in Kansas under many trying circumstances. On the frontier while fighting the pro-slavery sentiment and snakes and badgers, then later on through the Civil War, and after the Civil War, until on June 22nd, 1874, like a burst of sunshine the whole truth dawned on my mind, that I was gradually approaching a science by study, research, and observation that would be a great benefit to the world. (Still 1908, 85)

3. Frontier Education

In all things of nature there is something of the marvelous.

— ARISTOTLE

Still expounded in his autobiography:

> (11) Is the frontier a place to study science? our college-bred gentlemen

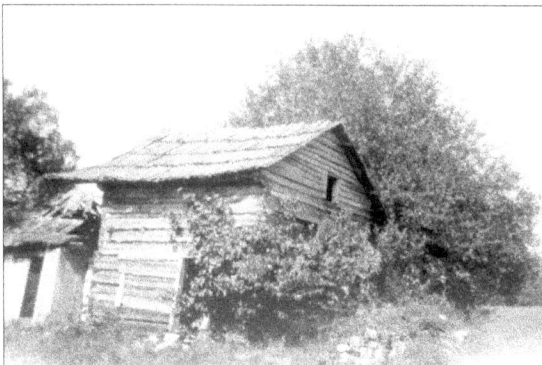

1.3 Photograph of Cabin in which A. T. Still was born in its original Virginia location. The cabin now exists in the Still National Osteopathic Museum. Courtesy Still National Osteopathic Museum, Kirksville, MO.

may ask. Henry Ward Beecher once remarked that it made very little difference how one acquired an education, whether it be in the classic shades and frescoed halls of old Oxford or Harvard, or by the fireside in the lonely cabin on the frontier. The frontier is a good place to get the truth. There is no one there to bother you. Beecher was then in mature years, and knew whereof he spoke. He had by the experience of a lifetime come to realize that a college education would not put good sense in a head where no brains existed.

The frontier is the great book of nature. It is the fountain-head of knowledge, and natural science is here taught from first principles. How does the scientist learn of the habits and manners of the animals that he wishes to study? By the observation of the animals. The old frontiersman knows more of the customs and habits of the wild animals than the scientist ever discovered. . . .

In the quiet of the frontier, surrounded by nature, I continued my study of anatomy with more zeal and more satisfactory results than I had at college. With no teacher but the facts of nature, and no classmates save the badger, coyote, and my mule, I sat down to my desk on the prairie to study over what I had learned at medical schools. With the theory firmly fixed in my mind that the "greatest study of man is man," I began with the skeleton. I improved my store in anatomical knowledge until I was quite familiar with every bone in the human body. The study of these bodies of ours has ever been

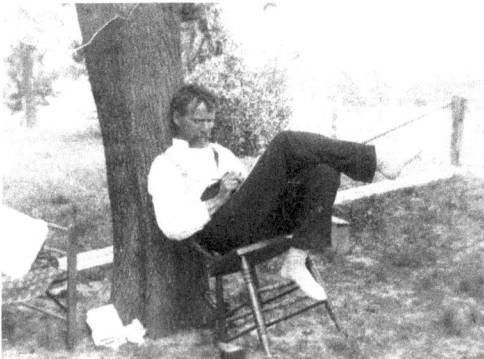

1.4 Dr. A. T. Still writing his autobiography at the Millard farm. Courtesy Still National Osteopathic Museum, Kirksville, MO.

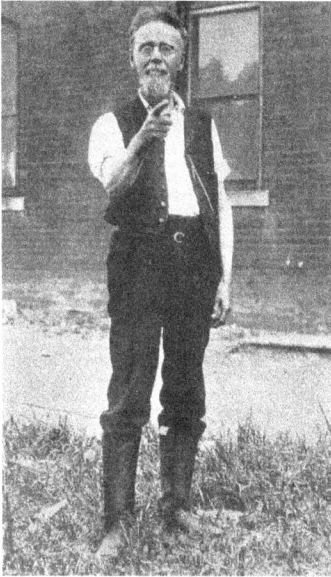

1.5 Dr. A. T. Still in a familiar attitude, ca. 1900. Courtesy Still National Osteopathic Museum, Kirksville, MO.

fascinating to me. I love the study and have always pursued it with zeal. Indian after Indian was exhumed and dissected, and still I was not satisfied. A thousand experiments were made with the bones, until I became quite familiar with the bony structure. (Still 1908, 85–86)

Dr. Homer E. Bailey gave the following characterization of Still: "He was a great student of nature and nature's laws, and never was happier than when he was astride an old log out in the woods . . ." Bailey went on to say, "Dr. Still was a man who personally disliked notoriety and advertisement, and when the clamor of the multitudes was so great in 1892 that he and his family could no longer heal the vast crowds that appeared before him, he began to teach others. He would hide himself away for days at a time, to obtain the quiet and rest which he so much needed in developing the science and building the school that he was then undertaking" (in Booth, 33).

Many said Still held a great likeness to his contemporary, Abraham Lincoln. In this regard,

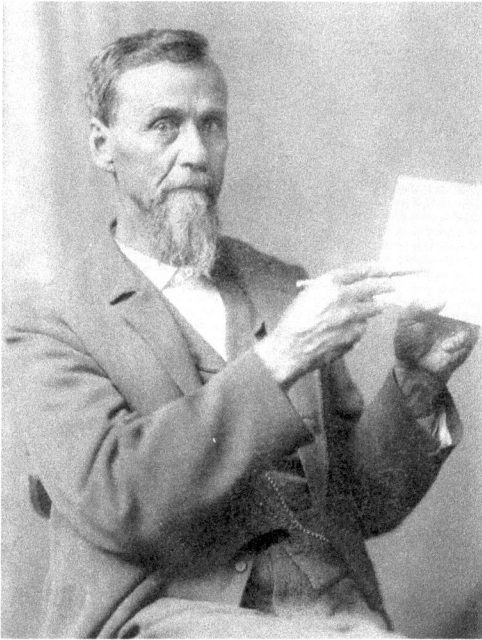

1.6   Dr. A. T. Still, 1898. Courtesy Still National Osteopathic Museum, Kirksville, MO.

Dr. J. H. Sullivan speaks thus of his first meeting with Dr. Still:

"My first meeting with Dr. A. T. Still occurred in 1894, through my wife's invalidism. We reached Kirksville and she went under treatment April 1, 1894.

"While waiting for our turn we noticed a remarkable appearing man dodging in and out of the rooms in his shirt sleeves, and we instinctively thought, this is the doctor we have come to see. He reminded me of the great emancipator, Lincoln, and many others have expressed the same thought; to complete the analogy, I heard him lecture after a few days and he said among other things: 'I helped free the colored man from slavery and am now engaged freeing the white man from slavery—slavery of drugs.' His results certainly have borne him out in this assertion . . .

"Dr. Still is not a university graduate in the higher sciences, nevertheless, many times have I heard him debate with scientific men, and never have I heard him at a loss for an answer, whether it were astronomy, electricity, mineralogy, or allied sciences, he invariably had his own peculiar solution of the question. In anatomy, vast as the subject is and intricate as well, Dr. Still has within him an almost supernatural acquaintance with the living model. The question never settled as to the function of the thyroid gland and the spleen, have been most satisfactorily explained by Dr. Still, as all students under him can bear witness." (in Booth, 34)

Both Lincoln and Still used the quietude of nature for study and reflection. The grass, forest, animals, and sky offered them the opportunity to contemplate and to observe reality.

4. Civil War and Drew's Grief

To the orthodox method of learning from books and specimens, Still added a more mysterious source for some of his acquired information. His ideas came from first-order knowledge, which he received *de novo* through contemplation and communion with spirit. Through stillness, Drew Still acquired, gathered, and ordered ideas that many other great thinkers have realized before and after him. Still's version

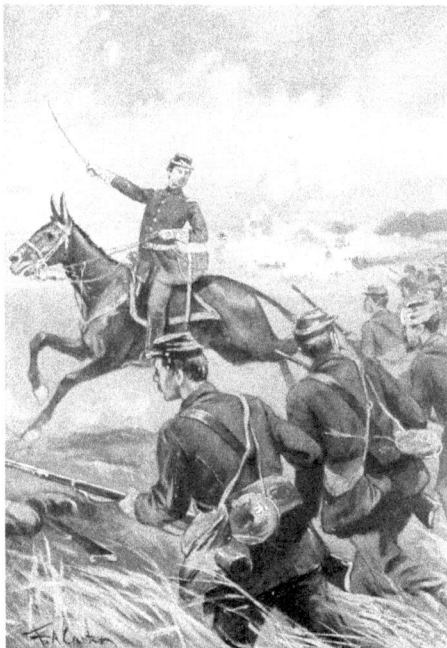

1.7 Painting depicting civil war battle (Osteopathy in Danger). Reproduced from *Autobiography of A. T. Still* 1897, p. 86.

of these timeless precepts was unique, fired by his personal tragedy and enlivened by his special talents.

Still wrote in his autobiography:

(11a) I might have advanced more rapidly in Osteopathy had not the Civil War interfered with the progress of my studies. We cannot say how a thing will appear until it is developed, and then we often find that the greatest good follows the greatest grief and woe, as you all know fire is the greatest test of the purity of gold . . . Not until my heart had been torn and lacerated with grief and affliction could I fully realize the inefficacy of drugs. Some may say that it was necessary that I should suffer in order that good might come, but I feel that my grief came through gross ignorance on the part of the medical profession.

It was in the spring of 1864; the distant thunders of the retreating war could be easily heard; but now a new enemy appeared. War had been very merciful to me compared with this foe. War had left my family unharmed; but when the dark wings of spinal meningitis hovered over the land, it seemed to select my loved ones for its prey. The doctors came and were faithful in their attendance. Day and night they nursed and cared for my sick, and administered their most trustworthy remedies, but all to no purpose . . . I had great faith in the honesty of my preacher and doctors then, and I have not lost that faith. God knows I believe they did what they thought was for the best . . .

It was when I stood gazing upon three members of my family,—two of my own children and one an adopted child,—all dead from the disease, spinal meningitis, that I propounded to myself the serious questions "In sickness has God left man in a world of guessing? Guess what is the matter? What to give, and guess the result? And when dead, guess where he goes?" I decided then that God was not a guessing God, but a God of truth. And all his works, spiritual and material, are harmonious. His law of animal life is absolute. So wise a God had certainly placed the remedy within the material house in which the spirit of life dwells. With this thought I trimmed my sail and launched my craft as an explorer. (Still 1908, 86–88)

5. Construction of Man

His search for the remedy that God placed "within the material house in which the spirit of life dwells" began in earnest as he recovered from his grief. Not only had he lost his three children in 1864 but, only five years before, in 1859, he had lost his first wife and two years before that, in 1857, his father had also succumbed. He also had to recover from nagging illnesses, including an inguinal hernia suffered when his horse fell on him at the battle of Westport during the Civil War. He began his search by continuing his study of anatomy, something he had started in his youth while dressing the animals that he skillfully hunted. He confirmed for himself that the anatomy revealed masterful handiwork. He studied the bones of many human specimens. He had a great supply because many people had died from an epidemic of cholera. Most were from the tribe of Shawnee Indians at the Wakarusa Mission in the Kansas Territory with whom he had lived and worked in the early 1850s as he had begun his study of medicine under the tutelage of his father, Abram, both a physician and a Methodist missionary.[17–20]

For him then, and for us now, bones served as *landmarks* by which one might detect structural aberrancies. They also provided *handles* to correct such distortions. The family of connective tissues, including bone, fabricates structures for the physical and energetic integrity of the organism. Bone distinguishes itself as the hardest connective tissue among all the rest, including fat, areolar tissue, muscles, tendons, ligaments, fasciae, and cartilage. To the astute observer, the connective tissues—bone being the prominent example—offer the opportunity to palpate structural asymmetries.

Once the thoughtful osteopathic physician discovers his or her patients' palpable asymmetries, she or he can infer from this infor-mation that potential dysfunctions of specific blood vessels, nerves, lymphatics, and viscera might also exist. Thus, the connective tissues provide structural clues for functional disturbances of the organs, clues that become more obvious via palpation of the relative positions and ranges of motion of firm bones. If, indeed, osteopathic philoso-phy bases itself on the structure-function interrelationship, then the position of bony landmarks and motions of joints must certainly be placed at the foundation of this philosophy and practice. The whole process of osteopathic palpatory diagnosis and treatment starts with the arrangement of the bones.

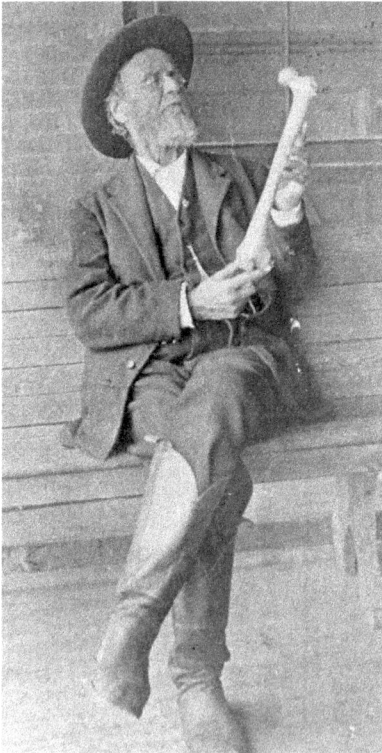

1.8 Dr. A. T. Still holding a femur. Courtesy Still National Osteopathic Museum, Kirksville, MO.

6. Still Coined "Osteopathy"

Still coined the term "Osteopathy" to denote the important role that osseous tissues play in the structure and function of the organism.

> (12) You wonder what Osteopathy is; you look in the medical diction-
> ary and find as its definition "bone disease." That is a grave mistake.
> Osteopathy is compounded of two words, osteon, meaning bone,
> pathos, pathine, to suffer. I reasoned that the bone, "Osteon," was the
> starting point from which I was to ascertain the cause of pathological
> conditions, and so I combined the "Osteo" with the "pathy" and had
> as a result, Osteopathy. (Still 1908, 184)

At times, he carried with him various skeletal specimens for study, in order to learn every attachment of muscle and ligament, every cross-ing or penetration of vessel and nerve, and every minute detail of the surface structure of each bone, including features that exhibit func-tional relationships with neighboring bones through joints and myo-fascial attachments. Photographs and personal accounts of Still during his early days in Kirksville depict him holding a bag of bones or an in-dividual bone, studying it. "Imagine one going about town, or strolling in the woods, dropping down perhaps upon a curbstone, taking a bone from among many hidden about his person, wholly oblivious of his surroundings, and studying it as if his whole future depended upon the exact origin or attachment of a muscle, perhaps mumbling to himself; and you will see Dr. Still" (Parker, in Booth, 38).

> (13) When I commenced this study I took the human bones and
> handled them, week in and week out, month in and month out, and
> never laid them down while I was awake for twelve months.
> (Still 1908, 269)

He required his early students to do as he did, to reach into a bag of bones and identify each one only by feel and distinguish from which side of the body it came. Such intimate knowledge of human construction via the minute inspection of these bones undoubtedly elevated Still to a level of awareness that few anatomists or clinicians have achieved. Applying this infinitesimal anatomical knowledge to problems related to health propelled Still, who was already prepared with uncommon skills, to a greater advantage than we as comparative osteopathic bystanders might conjecture (Still 1892, 20–21; Still 1908, 84–85; Trowbridge 1991, 128).

Still experienced, with his bony explorations, the holistic reality that comes to one who can see clearly, just as William Blake did when he wrote:

>to see a world
>in a grain of sand
>and a heaven
>in a wild flower,
>
>hold infinity
>in the palm
>of your hand
>and eternity
>in an hour.

Similarly, Still wrote:

(14) **To know all of a bone in its entirety would close both ends of an eternity.** (Still 1908, 152)

Hence, Still fittingly proclaimed *osteo-* (Gk. *osteon*) to be the root of the name of his new science, Osteopathy. He chose the suffix *-pathy* (Gk. *pathos*) to invoke a commonality with the names of other therapeutic systems of the time: homeo*pathy*, hydro*pathy*, allo*pathy*, and so on and to imply that, in Osteopathy, the bones perform a fundamental role in the identification of suffering (disease), as well as in its amelioration (therapeutics) (Still 1908, 184). Thus, in Osteopathy, the solid foundation on which we begin our discernment of the patient's root cause of suffering is by palpating bony relationships (*osteopathic palpatory diagnosis*), and further, one important way we address the alleviation of suffering by the management of bony alignment (*osteopathic manipulative treatment.*)

D. Somatic Dysfunction: Profession Defines Terms

After Still, the osteopathic profession accumulated decades of collective experience that spontaneously arose out of many centers as an empirical science. In an effort to collate clinical findings, to standardize terminology, and to consistently educate students at diverse colleges, the osteopathic profession established in 1953 a consensus regarding its philosophy.[21] Subsequently, the profession created the Educational Council on Osteopathic Principles (ECOP) to fulfill an ongoing effort for consistent word use and definitions at all the colleges of osteopathic medicine. To make more precise the common expression, "osteopathic lesion," ECOP created the term "somatic dysfunction": "Impaired or altered function of related components of the somatic (body framework) system: skeletal, arthrodial, and myofascial structures, and related vascular, lymphatic, and neural elements."[22]

Somatic dysfunction is that condition for which osteopathic manipulative treatment is therapeutic. The term "somatic dysfunction" formalized the collective clinical experience accumulated over several decades by the osteopathic medical profession about the adverse effects on physiology of asymmetry within the structural elements. The definition of "somatic dysfunction" reaches beyond just bony landmarks, those sentinels of structural asymmetry; it implicates additional aspects, just as Dr. Still did, of structurally based dysfunction, such as (1) impaired joint mechanics; (2) altered mechanics of the associated soft connective tissue (e.g., abnormal resting length of muscle, alteration of the tension of ligament, aberrant tension across fascia, strain in dura, and congestion in the extracellular matrix); (3) dysfunctions of arterial supply, venous and lymphatic drainage, and nerve conduction; and (4) changes in the tissues resulting from the foregoing to include tissue texture change (ropiness, thickness), swelling (edema), and/or tenderness of specific areas to touch. These elements of somatic dysfunction are often abbreviated TART (tissue texture change, asymmetry, restriction of motion, tenderness).

1. Soma and Viscera

Another element involves the relationship of these connective tissue findings to the function of organs.

> (15) Thus, we recognize the importance of a thorough acquaintance with the large and small fibers, ligaments, muscles, blood- and nerve-supply to all the organs. (Still 1892, 34)

Organ dysfunctions can be rooted in mechanical joint dysfunctions with their associated restrictions of fluid flows in blood and lymphatic vessels, aberrant neurological reflexes, abnormal congestion within the extracellular space, and pain. Still and the osteopathic physicians who followed him observed that somatic structure and organ function are related. To this day, this principle rests at the foundation of the profession's existence. Yet, for conventional medicine, the relationship of organ function and somatic structure is considered unproven, if not patently false. Let us discover the basics of this premise that divides two professions.

Osteopathic principles declare that if somatic dysfunction is present, organs may not be able to optimally perform, according to the following scenario. *Fluid movement* into lymphatic and venous capillaries that normally clear metabolic by-products and other pollutants from the cells and interstitial space is diminished in the case of somatic dysfunction. Palpable congestion, in the form of edema or induration, exists in the connective tissues as evidence of restricted fluid flow in the extracellular space. Such limitation of fluid flow increases the local concentration of products of metabolism and other acidic toxins. Such a localized polluted interstitium disturbs sensitive enzyme systems and cellular chemistry in the connective tissues and parenchyma.

Further, with somatic dysfunction comes the *irritation of nerve endings* that report to the central nervous system (CNS). Such nociception results from at least two influences: (1) chemical, for example, the accumulation of acidic and disabling toxins and/or changes in the concentrations of electrolytes, O_2, and H^+; and (2) mechanical, for example, the accumulation of fluids that restrict free and easy motion and/or proprioceptive distortion of the tissues. The nociceptive impulses originate from the connective tissues of the musculoskeletal system and/or the interstitium surrounding the organs.

Triggered by such nociceptive stimuli, impulses from the CNS adversely influence the activities of the viscera and connective tissues simultaneously through circuitry involving the sympathetic nervous system.[23] Whether the irritation originates in the organ or in the connective tissue, both can be (and usually are) *simultaneously* affected. This can be explained by the fact that afferent sensory nerves from both viscera and soma actually terminate within the same region of the dorsal horn of the spinal cord. Consequently, this nociceptive stimulus of the dorsal horn, from either a somatic or visceral source, equally generates an efferent signal that emanates from the ventral horn of the same region of the spinal cord. This efferent signal affects both the adjacent soma (paravertebral muscles, ligaments, and spinal joints) and distant organs because it passes through the sympathetic circuitry, which specifically innervates both soma and viscera from the same level of the cord. This simultaneous influence creates what is termed by osteopathic physicians a viscero-somatic or a somato-visceral reflex. The reflex is named first according to the tissue from which the stimulus originates and, second, for the tissue that is subsequently affected. Viscero-visceral and somato-somatic reflexes, extending from one level of the cord to another, also occur.[24–25]

A cycle of positive feedback establishes itself when, stimulated by such nociception, such an efferent signal produces:

1. Through motor nerves, an abnormally contracted muscle, which may consequently further irritate the nerve in question, which in turn exacerbates the contracted muscle.

2. A subsequent worsening of the joint mechanics, which decreases motion and consequently increases tissue turgor and/or pain with motion through mechanical and neurological influences, respectively, which in turn exacerbates the joint mechanics.

3. Through sympathetic nerves, a limitation of blood supply to compromise somatic tissues and/or a specific organ, which consequently reports alarm through increased rates of firing of afferent signals back to the cord, generating from the cord efferent signals that pass through the sympathetics to aggravate the limited blood supply.

4. A sick organ, which sends increased afferent signals to the cord whose motor and sympathetic output creates somatic dysfunction, which multiplies adverse afferent impulses to the cord, generating efferents from the cord that limit blood supply and aggravate the condition of the sick organ.

In the case of a primary musculoskeletal injury, afferents may stimulate through the sympathetic efferents a worsening of the already compromised health of the soma by diminished blood supply as well as the potential to reduce the health of a specific organ by a similar mechanism.

The scenarios described here are not comprehensive; nevertheless, they provide insight into the mechanisms of somato-visceral, viscero-somatic, somato-somatic, and viscero-visceral reflexes observed in the clinic. These scenarios show how the reflex arcs become established and, unless correct intervention is applied, can become chronic.

The foregoing explains the philosophical division between conventional medical and osteopathic physicians. Unless one has the skill and clinical experience to palpate the somatic dysfunction and to simultaneously obtain clinical information about its relationship to a specific organ dysfunction, one cannot speak with authority about whether somatic and visceral relationships actually exist. Physicians who have not received training in this discipline of osteopathic palpatory diagnosis cannot be expected to understand its characteristics or its value in diagnosis and treatment; as a result, they cannot competently comment on its utility or effectiveness. Although the technology does not exist to measure these reflexes, they are apparent on osteopathic palpatory exam, and osteopathic physicians have accumulated decades of clinical experience that speak volumes about the existence of these phenomena and the effectiveness of OMT in their amelioration.[26]

2. Osteopathic Manipulative Treatment

By what manner do osteopathic physicians address somatic dysfunction for the alleviation and prevention of suffering? Therapeutic intervention could theoretically be applied to the neurological circuitry, to the end organ, or to the somatic structure. Of course, the soma is much more accessible by palpatory means, both diagnostically and therapeutically, than any other component of the circuit. Thus, the interruption of the positive feedback loop is achieved by somatic input, that is, OMT. If one is able to correct an abnormally shortened muscle, for example, the whole process of somatic dysfunction unwinds itself. Restoring the muscle length to normal decongests the tissues and opens neural foramina to allow the afferents to quiet their previous hypertonic input to the cord. As the rate of firing of nerve impulses normalizes, shutting off the nociceptive input to the cord, the sympathetic output also normalizes and the vascular delivery of nutrients to end organs resumes a normal pace.

Counterstrain is an example of a technique directed at shortened muscles.[27] Other forms of OMT address other aspects of somatic dysfunction: joint mechanics (thrust, muscle energy, and functional techniques), fascial tension (myofascial, soft tissue, and cranial techniques), and organ dysfunction (visceral and cranial techniques). This list of techniques and the objects of treatment is not comprehensive but rather an example of the utility of various methods by osteopathic technicians.[28]

3. Osteopathic Palpatory Diagnosis

Aside from somatic pathophysiology and its therapeutic correction, osteopathic palpatory diagnosis offers the osteopathic physician important clues about impaired organ function and a significant diagnostic capability beyond standard medical diagnostic techniques. For example, osteopathic palpatory diagnosis helps the osteopathic physician differentiate among the causes of acute abdominal pain, under which circumstances diagnostic acumen can often be critical. By palpation of the spinal and paraspinal connective tissues, the skilled osteopathic physician can distinguish between acute cholecystitis and acute appendicitis, for example. Because the soma and viscera are related by a common innervation through sympathetic nerves and the dorsal horn of the same segment of the spinal cord, the osteopathic physician determines which organ is potentially compromised by the location along the spine of somatic findings of tissue texture, altered joint motion, asymmetry, and tenderness. Such somatic dysfunction is evidence of a potential viscero-somatic reflex (or a somato-visceral reflex.) These terms are modern advancements of Still's original observations.

> (16) I contend that the curing comes direct from the liberation of the interspinous and costal nerves, freed from the bone-pressure on the nerves of motion, sensation, and nutrition. (Still 1892, 39)

Beyond viscero-somatic and somato-visceral reflexes, deeper levels of palpatory skill (for example, such skill as one exercises in the discipline of visceral manipulation) offer to the well-trained individual the ability, through subtle palpation of the respiratory motion of the visceral organs, to directly distinguish exactly which organ has diminished function. The correction of the dysfunction is also within the purview of visceral manipulation.

These aforementioned concepts are standard in today's osteopathic literature and clinical practice. They outline the details about the constraints to optimal functioning that result from altered structure, that is, somatic dysfunction.[29] In summary, somatic dysfunction precisely defines Still's observations of disturbed somatic tissue mechanics relative to altered physiology of organs, vessels, and nerves. Although Still never created a nomenclature for structural findings relative to functional problems, somatic dysfunction is a modern advancement of Still's ideas, taking into account the modern information that has been added to the original information that Still passed down to us. We can assume that Still would have approved of this modern advancement because it allows clarity of comprehension and precision of practice. Thus, the structure-function interrelationship is fundamental to the modern osteopathic physician just as it was to Andrew Taylor Still.

II. LOOKING DEEPER AT OSTEOPATHY

A. Still Misapprehended

In the foregoing, we have concisely considered the concepts that osteopathic medicine routinely teaches as standard osteopathic philosophy and practice, yet we have omitted a significant part of Dr. Still's ideas. When we closely read his writings, it becomes clear that modern interpretations of osteopathic philosophy ignore concepts that were fundamental to Andrew Still as he developed Osteopathy. In fact, as we will see, the real power of his philosophy emanates from concepts that most of us have failed to reiterate. If we want to truly comprehend the fullness of the osteopathic philosophy, we must have before us all the aspects of Still's philosophy, including concepts that may have been forgotten. We presently will consider the ideas left out of today's standard curricula.

But first, why has the osteopathic medical profession misunderstood Drew Still? Clearly, only a comparative handful of people have ever achieved the knowledge and skill of Still. To acquire the ability and understanding that he did—even to conceive of Osteopathy—demanded a commitment of his being to intensive innovative investigation and ongoing profound reflection. His self-education was unusual not only in its length but also in its doggedness. He was a student of nature—geology, botany, and zoology—as well as of humans—anatomy, physiology, and chemistry. Burning grief and unrelenting searching by an inspired and driven spirit fired Still's process of learning. What's more, Still was gifted with skills of perception that few people would use as he did even if they happened to possess them. He displayed a genius-level rationality and an astounding intuition in obtaining the knowledge and insight from the moment that light pierced his perception at 10:00 am on June 22, 1874. Yes, he was truly inspired. These combined attributes and conditions in the life of one man were certainly unique and not easily duplicated by his osteopathic students and successors.

It is no wonder that others failed to fully apprehend Still's conception. E. R. Booth, PhD, DO, provided the following insight into the operation of Still's mind through his manner of speech: "The crowding in upon his mind of . . . thoughts . . . often give to his lectures, and even his conversation, an air of mysticism—of the supernatural. His ideas generally outrun his expression of them. His deepest thoughts often come to his mind with such rapidity and are uttered in such quick succession that the hearer may become dazed in attempting to follow him, and perhaps wonder whether there is a coherent principle underlying his expressions. A more thorough acquaintance with the Old Doctor and his methods of thought and work always convinced us that he had delved beyond our view, and that we had failed to comprehend his meaning" (Booth, 24).

As the quotation continues, Booth described Still's writing: "We often come across passages in his writings that are incomprehensible at first. A more thorough study of them or a few words of explanation often make such passages perfectly clear and reveal a mine of thought hitherto uncomprehended. To fully understand Dr. Still it is almost absolutely necessary to have a personal acquaintance with him. It is only by coming in close touch with him that his character becomes fully revealed. Often thoughts with which we are supposed to be familiar would be expressed in an unexpected moment. A single terse sentence apparently not connected with any thing preceeding [sic] or following would often be uttered and proclaim a profound truth" (Booth, 24).

Harry L. Chiles, DO, an early student and long-time secretary of the American Osteopathic Association and editor of the *Journal of the American Osteopathic Association,* gave the following account of his educational experience with Dr. Still: "It was difficult to follow his hand in some of his diagnoses and treatment. There was no hesitation, for he had a clear picture in his mind of the structures he was working with. None of us had that much knowledge and no one has matched his technic, nor his success. His instructions in technic were often over our heads, but his reasoning, his deductions, and his philosophy were of the greatest value" (in Hildreth 1938, 445).

Still is quoted as having said about his first class at the American School of Osteopathy "At the close of school I found that I had nothing but . . . bunglers, no anatomy—no osteopaths—time lost and nothing but imitators. I tried to get them to reason . . . but could not because of their lack of anatomical knowledge."[30] In an early edition of the *Journal of Osteopathy*, there is also reference to this first class. "One piece of advice was given to Still by Father Ryan, a Catholic priest, who admonished him, 'But few heads in your first class will ever be able to do honor to your great discovery and you must raise your standard of intelligence in your school or such a head will ruin the science and disgust the people before the world knows the merit of your discovery.' "[31] Still determined to continue with the effort of training others in Osteopathy, adapting the curriculum with each succeeding class and selecting them with care.

His students learned from him verbally and by demonstration, but were they truly able to perceive with their hands as he did? Were they able to obtain his experience, even if he succeeded in relating it? In this new discipline, Osteopathy, which simultaneously demanded intellectual exercise and palpatory perception, were his students able to integrate both of these and to apply them in the clinic? Were his students as driven, inspired, talented, and gifted as their mentor was? Were they as willing and able as Still to look beyond the ordinary means of acquiring information or past the ordinary manner of perceiving reality? Conversely, despite his gifts, was Still able to fully communicate what he intended? Furthermore, has time been true to his rendering of reality, to his "child, Osteopathy"? Has the translation from generation to generation been true?

From the confusion manifested today among osteopathic students, teachers, and practitioners about what Osteopathy is, it is clear that a common misunderstanding of A. T. Still persists.[32] It is also clear that this misapprehension may well have originated from his earliest efforts to pass on his wisdom. The context in which Dr. Still transmitted his thoughts played an equal role in confusing his hearers. He spoke of ideas that were new, and, in some circumstances, he spoke forcefully about concepts that were counter to the mainstream. Moreover, as we will see, his thoughts reached as far as the human mind can go, to the creation of the cosmos. Were his students at this time in human historical development prepared to hear these radical and complex notions? With all this in mind, and with his invitation to us to pluck the squirrel from the hole in the tree, a reevaluation of his ideas is in order. First, let us look at the impact of the misapprehension of Still's precepts on present-day osteopathic practice.

1. Professional Fallout

When modern osteopathic physicians come to fully comprehend Still's philosophy and its consequences, then and only then can each individual make an informed choice about his or her alignment with or commitment to the osteopathic philosophy and therefore to the osteopathic profession as a social movement. Because of the health-giving potential inherent in its practice, osteopathic medicine carries the obligation to firmly claim, to clearly state, and to powerfully promote its philosophy. Without such a staunch statement of philosophy and a committed cadre of physicians, the osteopathic medical profession loses its identity and its effectiveness as a cogent advocate of its unifying thesis and, at the same time, loses its opportunity to enlist its powerful healing philosophy. If medicine's primary goal is the alleviation of suffering and if osteopathic palpatory diagnosis and treatment achieve this goal when other means and therapies fail, then the osteopathic profession must promote its philosophy or fail to reach its potential and fulfill its promise to society.

Because of the power of the inherent truth and effectiveness of Still's philosophy, it naturally finds expression in other systems of health care, where it grows and prospers. As a result, today, we witness osteopathic concepts being promoted, sometimes by other names, by a variety of therapeutic disciplines and, in some cases, with more vitality, conviction, and persuasiveness than by Osteopathy.

2. Understanding Still

A deeper understanding of and a conviction about A. T. Still's ideas accrue to the diligent osteopathic explorer from at least two sources: palpation and mentation—that is, tactilely, through the experience of profound levels of osteopathic palpatory diagnosis and treatment, and intellectually, by thoroughly acquainting oneself with and deeply contemplating Still's writings. These two avenues, skill and knowledge, enhance and confirm each other. Through the development of skill in palpatory experience, we perceive evidence of Still's proclamations about inherent forces; reading Still's writings opens our minds to search for evidence of these inherent forces. To fully understand requires that, in many cases, a student of Still's philosophy must be committed to studying material beyond the standard curriculum of osteopathic medical school.

> (17) Some people have an idea that this science can be learned in five minutes. . . . If you can learn all of Osteopathy in four years I will buy you a farm and a wife to run it and boss you. (Still, in Booth, 42)

I recommend that anyone interested in learning the true healing potential that exists in the realm of Osteopathy explore the deeper levels of palpation as taught in the more subtle disciplines of osteopathic manipulative medicine, especially visceral and cranial manipulation.

(18) An intelligent head will soon learn that a soft hand and a gentle move is the hand and head that get the desired results.
(Still, in Booth, 40)

(19) One asks, how must we pull a bone to replace it? I reply, pull it to its proper place and leave it there. One man advises you to pull all bones you attempt to set until they pop. That popping is no criterion to go by. Bones do not always pop when they go back to their proper places nor does it mean they are properly adjusted when they do pop.
(Still 1910, 27)

For now, we leave the palpatory training to the preceptorship experience, limiting our discussion to the aspect of mentation; that is, we investigate Still's writings. We review Still's words and compare them with the modern definition of osteopathic medicine and with other authors and philosophies.

B. Missing Concept: Biogen

To complement today's standard curriculum of osteopathic philosophy, it is fundamentally important to include the concept biogen. In Chapter XI of *The Philosophy and Mechanical Principles of Osteopathy* (1892),* Still introduced the term "biogen." This book was not generally available until Still's descendents approved its rerelease in 1986. Still reconsidered the broad distribution of this book as soon as it was published. He recalled as many of the volumes as he could recapture and then shared the book with only those whom he carefully chose.

---

* There is some controversy about *Philosophy and Mechanical Principles of Osteopathy* being Still's first book. It may have been published in 1902, making this writing not his first attempt to articulate his ideas.

His family held the book in secret until his granddaughter, Mary Jane Denslow (with the approval of other family members, including Still's grandson, Charles E. Still, Jr.[33]), collaborated with two osteopathic physicians to republish it in its original form using photographic printing techniques. Speculation abounds as to the reason for Still's withholding of this information. Perhaps some of the information was too radical or inflammatory, or perhaps it gave away "proprietary secrets."

Much of the information for the present chapter comes from this book of Dr. Still. We recognize whole passages of this book restated in his other books, especially his *Autobiography* (1908) and *Philosophy of Osteopathy* (1899). Interestingly, in these other works he excluded the concept of biogen. Yet, as we see in the next chapter (see Chapter Two, Section I.B), G. D. Hulett, DO, the first professor of Principles and Practice of Osteopathy at the American School of Osteopathy, thoroughly discussed biogen and related ideas in his text, *Principles of Osteopathy* (1903).

What did Still mean by the term "biogen"? In *Webster's Third New International Dictionary* (1993) we find "biogen" defined as follows: "a hypothetical ultimate living unit of which cells are built up: Biophore." For "biophore," we discover the following definition: "the ultimate supramolecular vital unit . . . the basic building block of living structures." To grasp Still's meaning of this term, we must first understand what he meant by the term "life" and how it relates to what he called Celestial and Terrestrial life.

1. What Is Life?

To begin the in-depth exploration of Still's philosophy, we examine Still's conception about life, because it is basic to his concept of biogen.

(20) One has said, "Life is that calm force sent forth by Deity to vivify all nature." (Still 1892, 101)

(21) Life is that force sent forth by the Mind of the universe to move all nature, and apply all our energies to keep that living force at peace, by retaining the house of life in good form from foundation to dome. (Still 1892, 101)

Still indicated that life is a finely divided material substance, individualized from the all-moving force of Nature and given form by parent causes.

(22) What is Life? . . . It might be called an individualized principle of Nature. (Still 1892, 249)

(23) When matter passes beyond the degree of being atomized farther, then it is life. (Still 1892, 254)

(24) Life surely is a very finely prepared substance, which is the all-moving force of Nature, or that force that moves all nature from worlds to atoms. (Still 1892, 256)

(25) When matter ceases to be divisible, it then becomes a fluid of life and easily unites with other atoms, and is a mass or body of living matter and recrystallizes into the form given by the parent causes. (Still 1892, 254–255)

Still's concept of life correlated with his use of the term "biogen," the fundamental forces building the material of living structures. As we will discover, this "mass or body of living matter" is what Still called "biogen." Biogen is the primary expression of the life force in the material realm.

2. Life Invests Matter

Still described life investing itself with matter.

(26) If life is an individualized personage, as we might express that mysterious something, it must have definite arrangements by which it can be united and act with matter. (Still 1892, 249)

3. Life Is Motion

Dr. Still said that the only evidence of life is the motion it gives to material substance.

(27) We know life only by the motion of material bodies. (Still 1892, 255)

(28) We think it is not unreasonable to conclude that life is matter in motion. (Still 1892, 257)

In the following quotation, Still went so far as to imply that if life is to invest itself with matter, motion is imperative, or the union of the two will end.

(29) Life and matter can be united, and that . . . union cannot continue with any hindrance to free and absolute motion. (Still 1892, 250)

4. Celestial and Terrestrial

Two realms exist, the Celestial and Terrestrial* worlds, from which, by combining their unique properties, living beings originate.

---

* I capitalize "Celestial" and "Terrestrial" throughout the book to signify that I am using these terms in the manner that Still used them to refer to two different realms, one energetic, ethereal, spiritual, and mental and the other material, earthly, three-dimensional, and physical. He used these terms in conjunction with his descriptions of creation, in which he held that these two elements reciprocate to form an organism.

(30) In man's body have been prepared and united the two kinds of life, the celestial and terrestrial, and the result is man and beast. (Still 1892, 255)

Still then laid the ground for our understanding of how the triune nature of the human being derives from the two original realms of creation, the Celestial and Terrestrial worlds; how form and function manifest; and what biogen is.

(31) The celestial worlds of space or ether-life give forms wisely constructed in exchange for the use of the material substances. Reciprocity through the governments of the celestial and terrestrial worlds is ever the same, and human life, in form and motion, is the result of conception by the terrestrial mother from the celestial father. Thus, we have the union of mind, matter, and life, or man. (Still 1892, 251–252)

5. Human Is Triune

Still added the concept of Mind to the two elements of material substance and life force. He used the concept of spirit ("spiritual") in place of life in this next passage, as he did in various other places. He equated spirit with life.

(32) First, there is the material body; second, the spiritual being; third, a being of mind which is far superior to all vital motions and material forms, whose duty is to wisely manage this great engine of life. (Still 1892, 16–17)

Still wrote about the triune characteristic of the human in many ways. He indicated that the human being consists of material substance that is formed and vitalized by spirit and managed by mind. Thus, we see "Mind," "Matter," and "Motion,"* a phrase that has persisted through the decades of osteopathic lore.

In the next quotation, we could substitute the words "union of Mind, Matter, and spirit" or "Mind, Matter, and Motion" to give the same meaning. Still equated the terms "life," "motion," and "spirit."

> (33) Thus, we have the union of mind, matter, and life. . . .
> (Still 1892, 251–252)

Still performed a thought experiment to offer his readers an example of the three human qualities, Mind, Matter, and Motion, adding two of them individually to inert (dead) Matter (form).

> (34) When this great machine, man, ceases to move in all its parts, which we call death, the explorer's knife discovers no mind, no motion. He simply finds formulated matter, with no motor to move it, with no mind to direct it. Suppose the explorer is able to add the one principle motion; at once we would see an action, but it would be a confused action. Still he is not the man desired. There is one addition that is indispensable to control this active body, or machine, and that is mind. (Still 1892, 17)

First, we add Motion (life) to the still corpse and find we need control (Mind) over it in order to bring the form fully to normal human function. Therefore, Still believed that the governance of Mind is a critical component, in addition to Matter and spirit, for humans to be complete.

---

* I capitalize (1) "Mind," (2) "Matter," and (3) "Motion" throughout the book to signify that I am using these terms as Still used them to mean (1) the mind of God, consciousness directing a process; (2) material earthly substance; and (3) evidence of the life force or spirit in activity, emotion, behavior, metabolism, and life. He used these three terms when describing creation and the origins of humans.

6. Form and Motion

Still declared that the fundamental characteristic of life is Motion and that Motion endows the Matter that makes up the living human form through the agency of the "individualized principle" (life force). But from where does this endowment originate?

(35) **Thus man's body is a form given by celestial life to the terrestrial life.** (Still 1892, 255)

In this statement, Still indicated that the pattern of the form of humans originates from the Celestial world (Mind) and affects the Terrestrial world (Matter). Therefore, Still said that a pattern is drawn from the realm of Mind to serve as the plan for the material form.

(36) **Life terrestrial has motion and power; the celestial bodies have knowledge or wisdom.** (Still 1892, 251)

Here, Still categorized human qualities associating each with material and spiritual aspects. Motion drives the material form (Terrestrial), while control over that movement with wisdom comes from the Celestial world (Mind.)

These two components, Celestial and Terrestrial, come together and form life as in the following analogy.

(37) **The principle of the electric-light is the same as the principle of Osteopathy. It has two batteries composed of opposite chemicals; bring them together by action, and an explosion of light is produced.** (Still 1908, 252)

The combustion creates form, which demonstrates wisdom in its perfection.

> (38) We see the form of each world, [Celestial and Terrestrial] and call
> the united action biogenic life. All material bodies have life terrestrial
> and all [Celestial] space life, ethereal or spiritual life. The two, when
> united, form man. Biogen is the lives of the two in united action, that
> give motion and growth to all things. (Still 1892, 251)

In quotation (38), we close the circle and return to the term "biogen,"
the united action of Terrestrial and Celestial life. We have reviewed life:
life investing matter, life and Matter governed by Mind, and form and
Motion manifesting life by means of biogen. To summarize, human
form follows the pattern provided by Celestial life (Mind); is created
out of elements of the earth, or Terrestrial life (Matter); and is vitalized
by the life force (spirit), manifesting as form in Motion. Thus, biogen
is the fundamental concept of Still's philosophy. We discuss biogen further in the succeeding chapters.

7. Life Is Spirit

Just as he interchanged the terms "life" and "Motion," Still interchanged the words "life" and "spirit." In the following quotation, he
also used the word "physical" in place of "Matter" or "material" and the
word "spiritual" in place of "life" or "Motion."

> (39) The mind is asked to find the connection between the physical
> and the spiritual. (Still 1892, 249)

In *Webster's Third New International Dictionary* (1993), "spirit" is
defined as follows: "1: the breath of life: the animating or vital principle giving life to physical organisms." A further definition states, "the
active essence of the Deity serving as an invisible and life-giving or
inspiring power in motion." Discussions in this book regarding spirit
refer to the life force, the animating principle in humans, providing
power in motion. This is what Dr. Still meant by "spirit."

Vitalism. Dr. Still implied that life is a force, substance, or principle that vitalizes matter through a special relationship with it and creates an organization of the material substance to engender a form and a mechanism of function that manifests as motion. In philosophical terms, Still married several concepts, including mechanism, teleology, and vitalism. According to *Webster's Third New International Dictionary* (1993), "mechanism" is the doctrine that the processes of life are mechanically determined and explained by the laws of chemistry and physics, "teleology" is the doctrine that form is immanent in nature, that design in nature is determined by its utility or its Divine purpose, and "vitalism" is the doctrine that a living organism derives its functions from a vital principle.

Vitalism versus Mechanism. Often, philosophers refer to vitalism and mechanism as doctrines that oppose and exclude each other. That is, mechanism explains all activities of life by physics and chemistry to the exclusion of any mysterious vital force that cannot be explained in physical terms. Reductionistic and mechanistic approaches within science and medicine champion this view. However, practitioners of holistic disciplines often advocate vitalism, which for them subordinates physics and chemistry to the influence of the vital force; that is, any chemical or physical activity is ultimately attributable to the vital force.

Haller (1708–1777) may have been the first to claim that a vital force underlying all life phenomena is independent from chemical and physical laws.[34] Two recent reviews of vitalism by conventional scientists concluded that, despite discoveries of mechanisms of physics and chemistry that explain phenomena that were previously attributed to vitalism, nevertheless vitalism cannot be disproved and may, in fact, underlie the mechanisms.[35-36] In other words, the mechanisms of physics and chemistry may simply be the methods that spirit uses in biological systems to carry out the impetus for life that generates from Creator. Apparently, Still's opinion about what he referred to as life was consistent with this view. To summarize Still's previous quotations regarding the life force, we could say that life (vital force or spirit) interacts with matter (disorganized, earthly, material substance) and creates form (matter in the form of an organism) and motion (physics and chemistry).

C. Spirit and Osteopathy

The modern definition of osteopathic medicine that one sees includes the word "spiritual." Yet of all the adjectives used in this modern definition to characterize osteopathic medicine, spiritual is the single concept that remains relatively unexplored in the osteopathic classroom and clinic. All the other disciplines included in the modern definition—medicine, surgery, behavior, chemistry, physics, and biology—are taught to the depth that the teacher deems appropriate and that the student needs and desires. We routinely teach and practice all these disciplines as osteopathic educators and clinicians, with one exception: spirit.

In the "tenets of osteopathic medicine" developed by an ad hoc committee of the AOA in 2002, we find the term "spirit" mentioned; however, in the "principles for patient care" there is no provision for integrating spirit into treatment or the daily practice of osteopathic medicine.

1. Spirit Was Fundamental

Spirit was, in fact, fundamental for Still's philosophy of medicine. In *The Philosophy and Mechanical Principles of Osteopathy* (1892), Still opened with this sentence:

(40) **I quote no authors but God and experience.**

Here, in the first sentence of this important book, Still indicated that Osteopathy is based on God. He clarified that he referenced no other texts and that therefore the science of Osteopathy originated with him. He implied that he based his philosophy on inspiration (God) and diligent observation (experience.) He also said:

> (41) **God is the Father of Osteopathy, and I am not ashamed of the child of His mind. (Still 1908, 254)**

2. Study of the Real Spiritual Man

Dr. Still studied the "real spiritual man."

> (42) **Having spent many years of my life in the study of the anatomy of the physical man, of his bony framework and all thereunto attached, I have also tried to acquaint myself with the real spiritual man. (Still, in Booth, 18)**

As Dr. Truhlar wrote in 1950: "Many of the older Doctors expressed the feeling, that there must be a greater 'spiritual understanding' of Osteopathy in the profession. Dr. Andrew Taylor Still had this understanding of the human body as created by the 'Divine Architect', many of the older men and the successful ones in our profession have this 'spiritual concept'."[37]

Today, we can continue Still's search for the "real spiritual man." We can develop the idea of spirit as it relates to osteopathic medicine in a way that is similar to the manner in which the profession developed the concept of somatic dysfunction. We can examine Still's meaning in his writing and then apply modern advancements (or ancient ones, as the case may be) to flesh out a relevant interpretation for today. We can even provide the practitioner with a definition and a descriptive name for the expanded concept, as ECOP did for the idea of the "osteopathic lesion," which then became "somatic dysfunction." This discourse is an early attempt at this task. I hope that the task will not end here with this effort and with this author.

3. Spirit versus Religion

At this point in the book, we must clearly differentiate between spirituality and religion. In his autobiography, Still distinguished between the two:

> (43) I do not understand a preacher's business. I have not made a study of the Bible for that purpose; but the knowledge I have gained of the construction of man convinces me of the supreme wisdom of the Deity. (Still 1908, 306)

In this statement, Dr. Still confirmed that, for him, the design of the human organism provides convincing evidence of a supreme being. Further, he implied that his philosophy is not religious; rather, it is spiritual, honoring spirit as a basic influence in the construction of humans.

Carol Trowbridge, in her biography *Andrew Taylor Still, 1828– 1917,* claims that Still "was outspoken in his disbelief in a personal God and his distaste for all church organizations" (120). His father, in addition to being a physician, was a Methodist minister and Christian missionary, so obviously Drew was raised in a religious home. He read medicine under his father's tutelage at the Wakarusa Shawnee Indian Mission in the Kansas Territory. Nevertheless, A. T. Still claimed to "not understand a preacher's business," divorcing himself from religion, demonstrating his characteristic tendency to rebel against convention.

Trowbridge said that his dabbling in spiritualism and in evolutionary theories further marred his relationship with the clergy. Trowbridge went on to say, "He told a preacher that when he was 'through the study of the anatomy of man, and the laws that govern animal life, he would try a few thousand years in the juvenile class of the school of the infinite.' When the preacher denounced him as sacrilegious, Still answered that the 'divine' law was good enough for him. Still's use of the word 'divine' to describe what many preachers in 1874 considered

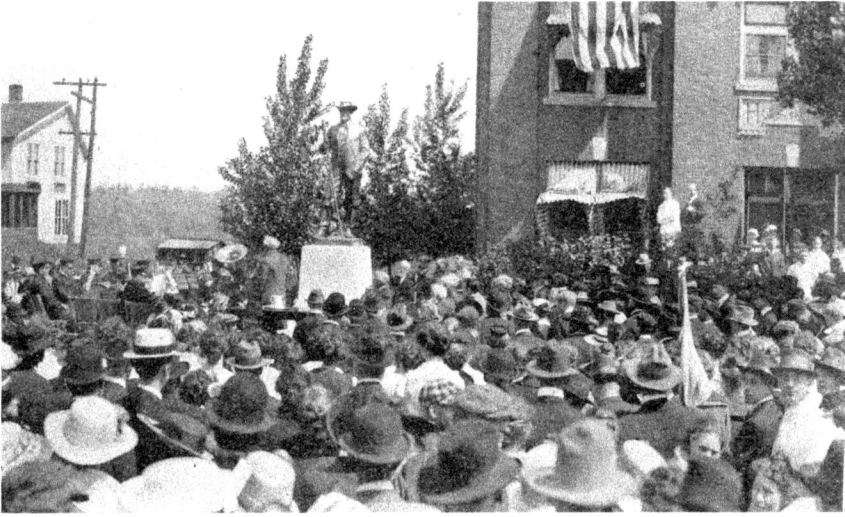

1.9 Dedication of A. T. Still's statue in front of ASO Hospital, May 23, 1917. Courtesy Still National Osteopathic Museum, Kirksville, MO.

to be an atheistic idea [evolution] was worrisome." Yet it is clear that Still had a strong belief in God. He said:

(44) For the last twenty-five years my object has been to find one single defect in all nature, to find one single mistake of God. But I have made a total failure in this respect. (Still, in Booth, 15–16)

The inscription beneath his statue in the courthouse square in Kirksville, Missouri reads:

(45) THE GOD I WORSHIP DEMONSTRATES ALL HIS WORK. DR. A. T. STILL.

"His religion, judged from the philosophical standpoint, might be considered pantheistic. Practically, Dr. Still is a spiritualist. Knowing as he does the frauds that have been practiced in the name of religion, and the misapprehension of most people concerning those who believe as he does, he has never forced his beliefs on any one" (Booth, 16).

It is clear from this description of Still's attitudes that he was not oriented to conventional religion. He used spirit as the source of his cosmology. Spirit, not religion, was fundamental to Still's philosophy of medicine. Let us move to the next set of conclusions to be drawn from a spiritual basis of this medical philosophy, Osteopathy.

D. Derivatives of Mind, Matter, and Motion

The consequences of biogen, that is, form in motion or the product of the union of life with matter, are many. Some of the most prominent examples of these are considered today to be the basic precepts of osteopathic philosophy.

1. Holism

Webster's Third New International Dictionary defines "holism" as follows: "the philosophic theory first formulated by Jan C. Smuts that the determining factors in nature are wholes (as organisms) which are irreducible to the sum of their parts." In other words, according to these principles, reductionism cannot explain the behavior of the whole. Smuts, a South African philosopher, coined the term "holism" in 1925 to counter the trend toward reductionism. He said we could only know the individual in context. One must study his or her social, environmental, and vocational aspects. That which exemplifies the unity of the system brings an important understanding to the function of the system.

Still also wrote about holism as a product of Mind, Matter, and Motion.

(46) The human form indicates an object . . . It is constructed as a hieroglyphical representation of all beings and principles interested physically or mentally in the production of worlds, with their material

forms, their living motions, and their mental governments.
(Still 1892, 27)

(47) I can hand this subject to you as a science that can be as plainly
demonstrated as the science of electricity. I find in man a miniature
universe. I find matter, motion, and mind. (Still 1908, 333)

Still implied that the human form, a hieroglyphical representation, comes from an image of something prior. This preexisting image
of the hieroglyph (body) is what Still repeatedly referred to in his writings as "the plans and specifications" for the body. This blueprint (to
substitute a modern term) for the structure of the body comes from a
spiritual (Celestial) source because, as Dr. Still said, it is a "representation of all beings and principles interested . . . in the production of
worlds." In other words, it comes as an image of God (or gods, if one is
pantheistic). Thus, the human form is a representation, in microcosm,
of the All-That-Is, the macrocosm (Mind).

(48) All patterns for all things are imitations of what is found in the
constructed being, man. We see in man, as we comprehend it, the attributes of Deity. We see the result of the action of mind, therefore a
representation of the Mind of all minds. We find in the solar system
motion, without which no universe can exist. (Still 1908, 259)

(49) I feel able through Osteopathy to look at Saturn and see it as a
small corpuscle of blood in the body of the great universe. When I
look at the earth, and the moon, and the solar system, I find that the
directing Mind has numbered every corpuscle in the solar system,
and each one of them comes in its round on time—no mistakes.
(Still 1908, 228)

These declarations from Still are holistic: A being functions as a whole, and each part of a being represents the whole being. The whole, in turn, represents a still larger whole. Still's hieroglyph (body) represents a larger whole (worlds) and, in turn, the larger whole reciprocates to provide the image for the body (hieroglyph).

> (31a) The celestial worlds of space or ether-life give forms wisely constructed in exchange for the use of the material substances. Reciprocity through the governments of the celestial and terrestrial worlds is ever the same, and human life, in form and motion, is the result of conception by the terrestrial mother from the celestial father. Thus, we have the union of mind, matter, and life, or man. (Still 1892, 251–252)

The previous quotation is repeated here for clarity and to reinforce its meaning. It describes, according to Still, the manner by which the Terrestrial and Celestial worlds reciprocate, the Celestial using material substance and the Terrestrial using an energetic blueprint to create a living form.

2. Health

Returning the structure and function of the body to a state that existed prior to trauma or illness defines the process of healing. According to *Webster's Third New International Dictionary,* health is a state of being whole, vital, flourishing, and functionally balanced. It is harmony.

> (50) What is harmony but health? It takes harmony of every nerve, vein, and artery in every part of the body. (Still 1908, 248)

Some have defined health as the mere absence of disease. Still said that disease is not the issue; rather, health is inherent within the living organism, throughout, in the tissues, nerves, and blood.

> (51) To find health should be the object of the doctor. Anyone can find disease. (Still 1892, 72)

3. Disease Is an Effect

There are no causes within the observable world. As we shall demonstrate, the observable world is a world of effects.

— DAVID HAWKINS

Osteopaths must look for the *cause* of disease in Nature.

(52) Sickness is an effect caused by the stoppage of some supply of fluid or quality of life . . . He conquers the disease by knowing how to apply the principles of this science along the lines of sensation, motion, and nutrition . . . An Osteopath is taught that nature is to be trusted to the end. (Still 1908, 252)

(53) What we meet with in all diseases is dead blood, stagnant lymph, and albumen in a semi-vital or dead and decomposing condition all through the lymphatics and other parts of the body, brain, lungs, kidneys, liver, and fascia. The whole system is loaded with a confused mass of blood that is mixed with unhealthy substances that should have been kept washed out by lymph. (Still 1892, 68)

4. Healing Applies Divine Law

The perfection of humans, made by the God of Nature, verified for Still humans' inherent ability for self-healing. According to Still, there is a characteristic of God evident in the restoration of an individual to a state of health. Healing involves spirit. If healing returns the organism toward balance, its original structure and function, then the organism returns toward perfection, that state in which spirit first manifests in material form as biogen. Still confirmed in clear terms that healing is divine when he said:

(54) It is our fortune at this time to raise our heads above the muddy

waters far enough to have a glimpse of the law that we choose to call Divine law. That law we use in healing. (Still 1908, 226)

Still said that he had traced the "Divine Law" that we use in healing.

> (55) We have traced it by reason, by philosophy, under the microscope, in the light and in the dark; and we hear a response. That response is so intelligent, its answer is so correct that a man is forced to believe there is knowledge behind it. (Still 1908, 226)

Stephen Paulus, DO, put it this way, "Health originates from the Divinity, or the Divine Inspiration that gives us life. When A. T. Still said, *'I love my fellow man, because I see God in his face and in his form,'* he was seeing the Original Cause in each patient he treated osteopathically!"[39]

5. Health from Nature

The source of health, according to Still, is "Nature."

> (56) In Nature we look for good machines in form and action. We have learned to know that Nature does no imperfect work, but, on the other hand, does its work to perfection. . . . (Still 1892, 22)

6. Nature Is Perfect

Because the God of Nature's wisdom is perfect and creates the human form, so too is the human form perfect.

> (57) I can trust the principles that I believe are found in the human body. I find what is necessary for the health, comfort, happiness of man, the passions, and all else. Nothing is needed but plain, ordinary diet and exercise. We find all the machinery, qualities, and principles that the Architect intended should be in man. Therefore, let me work

with that body, from the brain to the feet. It is all finished work, and is trustworthy in all its parts. (Still 1908, 248)

(58) The result is faultless perfection, because the earth-life shows in material forms the wisdom of the God of the celestial. (Still 1892, 251)

(59) Let us study man, who was made after wonderful plans and specifications, and when was completed was pronounced not only good, but very good, by that scrutinizing Inspector who makes all and omits nothing. (Still 1892, 14)

7. Man the Machine

"An All-wise Creator was the designer of our bodies as well as the author of our spirits, and . . . the human body is, therefore, a perfect machine" (Booth, 49).

(60) As motion is the first and only evidence of life, by this thought we are conducted to the machinery through which life works to accomplish the results as witnessed in "motion". (Still 1892, 250)

For Still, life is primary to the machinery, not the other way around. Once we accept the principle that motion manifests life, we proceed to examine the physical form that is found to be moving. But first comes the motion, the function.

(61) I began to look at man. What did I find? I found myself in the presence of an engine—the greatest engine that mind could conceive of. (Still 1908, 262)

8. Adjust Machine's Parts

In his writings, Still identified the salient aspects of the human—Mind, Matter, and Motion—and he then went on to develop a means by which one might engage and reorder the Matter (structure) and Motion (function) of the body. His concern was to permit health to take over by adjusting all parts back to normal.

> (62) An Osteopath is only a human engineer, who should understand all the laws governing his engine and thereby master disease.
> (Still 1908, 253)

> (63) Osteopathic practice [is] curing diseases by skillful readjustment of the parts of the body that have been deranged by strains, falls, or any other cause that may have removed even a minute nerve from the normal, although not more than the thousandth of an inch. He sees cause in a slight anatomical deviation for the beginning of disease. (Still 1892, 18)

9. Body's Own Remedies

Still wrote in his *Autobiography* that remedies exist within the health-giving nature of the tissues themselves. If the body is a Divine representation of perfection, then it follows that health is inherent within the body.

> (64) Believing that a loving, intelligent Maker of man had deposited in his body in some place or throughout the whole system drugs in abundance to cure all infirmities, . . . they can be administered by adjusting the body in such a manner that the remedies may naturally associate themselves together . . . God or nature is the only doctor whom man should respect. Man should study and use the drugs compounded in his own body. (Still 1908, 88–89)

10. Fascia

Still's concept that the terrestrial life unites with the celestial life to produce biogen, human form in motion, is consistent with his idea that the terrestrial aspect is relatively inert and that for it to move with living activity it must have the vivifying influence of the Celestial aspect. The material aspect of the human form must be activated by life (Still 1892, 257).

A. Spirit in the Material Man.

(65) The fascia . . . is the "material man." (Still 1892, 65)

(66) Life enters the forest of flesh as man. (Still 1892, 258)

(67) The soul of man, with all the streams of pure living water, seems to dwell in the fascia of the body. (Still 1892, 61)

(68) I want to draw the mind of the reader to the fact that no being can be formed without material, a place in which to be developed, and with all forces necessary for the work. (Still 1892, 114)

B. Nourishment. The fascia, with its nerves and blood, nourishes the body.

(69) [Fascia] gives nourishment to all parts of the body. Its nerves are so abundant that no atom of flesh fails to get nerve- and blood-supply therefrom. (Still 1892, 60)

(70) The cord throws out millions of nerves to all organs and parts which are supplied with the elements of motion and sensation. All these nerves go to and terminate in that great system, the fascia. (Still 1892, 64)

C. Disease Germinates. The fascia is not only the dwelling place of the soul (life), but also where the seeds of disease germinate.

(71) He has seen in the fascia the framework of life, the dwelling-place in which life sojourns. . . . He feels that he there can find all disturbing causes of life, the place in which diseases germinate and develop the seeds of sickness and death. (Still 1892, 61)

(72) All organs have coverings of this substance, though they may have special names by which they are designated. I write at length of the universality of the fascia to impress the reader with the idea that this connecting substance must be free at all parts to receive and discharge all fluids, and to appropriate and use them in sustaining animal life, and eject all impurities, that health may not be impaired by dead and poisonous fluids. A knowledge of the universal extent of the fascia is imperative, and is one of the greatest aids to the person who seeks the causes of disease. (Still 1892, 61)

(73) Just as surely at one place as the other . . . the poisonous effects are carried along to every fiber of the whole body by the nerves and fibers of the fascia. (Still 1892, 62)

11. Nerves and Blood

Dr. Still believed that the necessary elements for life were not only represented by biogen but were also replenished by the nerves and blood. Still noted the various functions provided by nerves.

(74) Now we must reason, if we succeed in relieving lungs, that all kinds of nerves are found in them. The lungs move, thus you find motor nerves; they have feeling, thus the sensory nerves; they grow by nutrition, thus the nutrient nerves. They move by will, or without it; they have a voluntary and involuntary system. (Still 1892, 63)

The whole body possesses the life force, and the blood is one of the carriers of it.

(75) They are surprised to find that the Great Architect has put in their proper places within man all of the processes of life. . . . He is surprised . . . to find the eternal truths of Deity permeating his whole makeup. . . . The wisdom of Nature's architect is found in every drop of your blood. (Still 1908, 330)

The life force, generated from the union of the Celestial and the Terrestrial, is delivered by blood that is under the control of the nerves.

(76) Harmony only dwells where obstructions do not exist. . . . Life and matter can be united, and that union cannot continue with any hindrance to the free and absolute motion. Therefore his [the osteopath's] duty is to keep away from the track all that will hinder the complete passage of the forces of the nervous system, that by that power the blood may be delivered and adjusted, to keep the system in normal condition. (Still 1899, 197)

Blood and nerves convey vital forces.

(77) The operator is supposed to come into this important battle, where local life is to be saved by increasing the vital force and supplying pure and healthy blood. He should halt and establish himself for observation as a seeker of the cause of this local delay in circulation, venous or arterial, and in the nerve-action, because in these three are the powers to supply the vital fluids and remove the exhausted. Vital forces must have access to the veins and arteries going to and from this irritating overplus of blood, fluids, and gases that are occupying the spaces in the skin, membranes, lymphatics, fascia, superficial and deep. (Still 1892, 82)

Blood fights infection.

(78) I began to realize the power of Nature to cure after a skillful correction of conditions causing abnormalities had been accomplished so as to bring forth pure and healthy blood, the greatest known germicide. With this faith and by this method of reasoning, I began to treat diseases by osteopathy as an experiment; and notwithstanding I obtained good results in all diseases, I hesitated for years to proclaim my discovery. But at last I took my stand on this rock, where I have stood and fought the battles and taken the enemy's flag in every engagement for the last twenty-nine years. (Still 1892, 10)

Poor circulation is responsible for many diseases.

(79) Take scrofula, consumption, eczema, every one of them. There is a broken current, an unfriendly relation existing between the capillaries of the veins and the arteries. (Still 1908, 280)

(80) The osteopath's first and last duty is to look well to a healthy blood- and nerve-supply. (Still 1892, 121)

12. Lymphatics

Still called the lymphatics the universal system of irrigation (1892, 65).

(81) We lay much stress on the uses of blood and the powers of the nerves, but have we any evidence that they are of more vital importance than the lymphatics? (Still 1892, 65)

(82) After beholding the lymphatics distributed along all nerves, blood-channels, muscles, glands, and all the organs of the body, from the brain to the soles of the feet, all loaded to fullness with watery liquids, we certainly can make but one conclusion as to their use,

which would be to mingle with and carry out all impurities of the body, by first mixing with the substances and reducing them to that degree of fineness that will allow them to pass through the smallest tubes of the excretory system, and by that method free the body from all deposits of either solids or fluids, and leave nourishment. (Still 1892, 65–66)

(83) Finer nerves dwell with the lymphatics than even with the eye . . . No atom can leave the lymphatics in an imperfect state and get a union with any part of the body. There the atom obtains form and knowledge of how and what to do. (Still 1892, 66)

(84) The lymphatics are closely and universally connected with the spinal cord and all other nerves, and all drink from the waters of the brain. (Still 1892, 66)

13. Cerebrospinal Fluid

Still declared that the cerebrospinal fluid contains the life force, as well.

(85) Thus all things else may be in place and in ample quantities and yet fail, because the power is withheld and there is no action for want of brain-fluids with their power to vivify all animated nature. (Still 1892, 53)

(86) A thought strikes him that the cerebro-spinal fluid is one of the highest known elements that are contained in the body, and unless the brain furnishes this fluid in abundance, a disabled condition of the body will remain. He who is able to reason will see that this great river of life must be tapped and the withering field irrigated at once, or the harvest of health be forever lost. (Still 1892, 44–45)

E. Opposed to Drugs

For Still, the flow of health is permitted by free-flowing structure. Health is immanent within biogen. Structural blockages impede the flow of health. Chemical interference in the form of drugs, especially those whose effects are poisonous, also causes an impediment to the free flow of health within the tissues. Still implied that, if one administers foreign substances, one assumes to know better than God.

> (87) **Either God is God, or He is not. Osteopathy is God's law, and whoever can improve on God's law is superior to God Himself.**
> (Still 1908, 224)

Instead, he directed his students to rely on the drugs native to the body. These inherent substances can be

> (88) **administered by adjusting the body in such a manner that the remedies may naturally associate themselves together.**
> (Still 1908, 89)

Yet, in the vein of denying the use of drugs, he said:

> (89) If you think an unerring God has made all those necessary preparations, why not so assert yourself, and stand upon that ground? . . . If in the human body you can find the most wonderful chemical laboratory mind can conceive, why not give more of your time to that subject, in order that you may obtain a better understanding of its workings? . . . Is it not ignorance of the workings of this divine law that has given birth to the foundationless nightmare now prevailing to such an alarming extent all over civilization, that a deadly drug will prove its efficacy in warding off disease in a better way than has been prescribed by the intelligent God who has formulated and combined

life, mind, and matter in such a manner that it becomes a connecting link between a world of mind and that element known as matter? Can a deep philosopher do otherwise than conclude that Nature has placed in man all qualities for his comfort and longevity? Or will he drink that which is deadly, and cast his vote for the crucifixion of knowledge? (Still 1892, 71)

He attributed his move away from the poisonous drugs used in those days for "doctoring" to J. M. Neal, a medical doctor of Edinburgh, Scotland, who said, "drugs were a bait for fools." Still quoted Neal further when he went on to say, "Nature was a law capable of

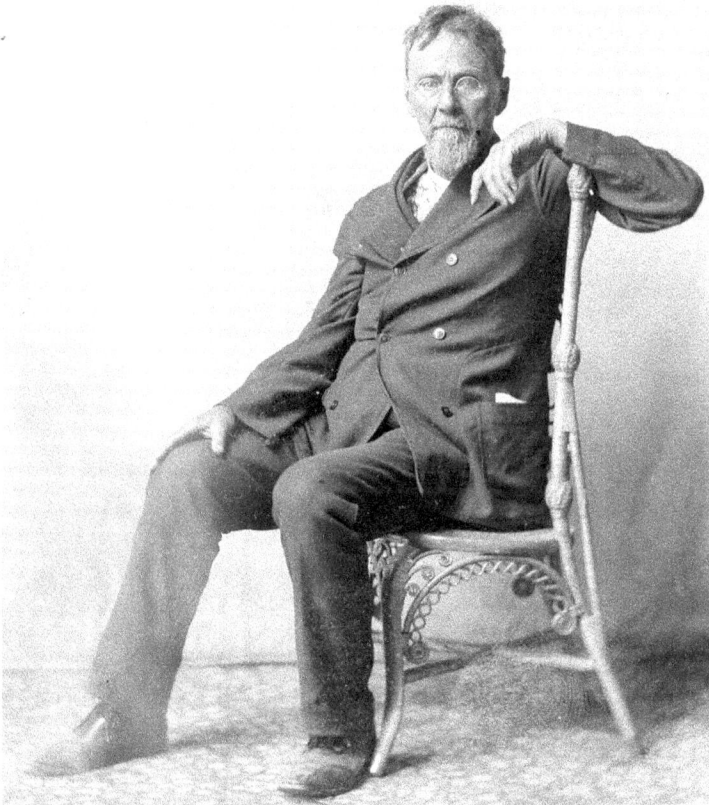

1.10 Dr. A. T. Still, 1903. Courtesy Still National Osteopathic Museum, Kirksville, MO.

vindicating its power to cure" (Still 1892, 9–10). Still and Neal favored the influence of Nature over that of the drugs of their day. In reference to Colonel Abbott, he said:

> (90) I began to give reasons for my faith in the laws of life as given to men, worlds, and beings by the God of Nature, in April, 1855. I thought the swords and cannons of Nature were pointed and trained upon our systems of drug doctoring. (Still 1892, 9–10)

F. What Is an Osteopath?

> (91) An up-to-date osteopath must have a masterful knowledge of anatomy and physiology. He must have the brains in osteopathic surgery, osteopathic obstetrics, and osteopathic practice . . . An osteopath answers questions by his learning. He proves what he says by what he does . . . He proceeds as a mechanic. (Still 1892, 18–20)

> (92) Surgery . . . is to be used as often or as much as wisdom finds it necessary in order to give relief and save life and limb when all evidence with facts shows that blood cannot repair the injuries. . . . Osteopathy is surgery from a physiological standpoint. The osteopathic surgeon uses "the knife of blood" to keep out "the knife of steel," and saves life by saving the injured or diseased limbs and organs of the body by reduction, in place of removing them. (Still 1892, 34–35)

> (93) I want to drag both of your feet out of the ruts of allopathy, and place your hands upon the handle of the pump and get some water from the lymphatics, the cellular system of the lungs, or any other place in the human body, set the excretories all to work. (Still 1892, 83)

> (94) I constantly urge my students to keep their minds full of pictures

of the normal body. (Still 1892, 9)

(95) If you go out thinking that Osteopathy is a good aid to medicine, you are using the words of incompetency.[40]

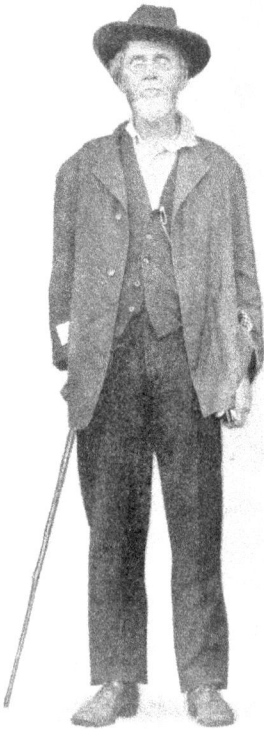

1.11 A. T. Still, ca. 1913. Courtesy Still National osteopathic Museum, Kirksville, MO.

III. SUMMARY

Dr. Still believed that healing originates from within the individual because of the fulfillment of spirit's potential to create form and function. Some deviation from the original design of the form, resulting from trauma or disease, interferes with spirit's ability to accomplish this fulfillment, and this condition requires some assistance from the outside to correct. Restoring the distortion of the structure toward normal liberates spirit to reassume its role of providing health. The following are summary statements of Still's philosophy that record the basic truths of Nature as they apply to healing.

1. Mind, Matter, and Motion compose creation.

2. Mind is the element of the Celestial realm.

3. Matter is the element of the Terrestrial realm.

4. The Celestial and Terrestrial realms reciprocate to produce form and Motion, biogen.

   a. Mind provides the patterns for material forms.

   b. Matter provides the material substance to manifest the forms.

   c. Motion is evidence of life existing in Matter. Matter without Motion is dead.

5. Mind demonstrates Creator's wisdom by perfection and Motion of form.

6. Life, or spirit, is a fine substance that invests itself with and vivifies Matter.

7. Biogen, Matter in Motion, is the primary living manifestation of spirit.

8. Health, spirit in action, is inherent in biogen.

9. Disease is a distortion of the form, of Mind's pattern, obstructing spirit.

10. Healing is a divine act, liberating spirit, restoring Motion to Matter.

11. Fluids—cerebrospinal fluid, blood, and lymph—contain and transport spirit.

12. Electrical and chemical energy are manifestations of spirit.

13. The brain is a dynamo, storing and discharging electricity via nerves.

14. The heart receives spirit and distributes it through arteries and nerves.

15. Arterial blood and nerves build, repair, and maintain the organism.

16. The fascia is the "material man," whose spirit resides in its fluids.

17. The body is a hologram, representing the macrocosm.

18. Adjusting connective tissues optimizes the activity of spirit and healing.

19. Drugs from within the body are to be trusted, not those from without.

20. The use of these principles provides a natural and rational basis for healing in the practice of medicine.

It is clear from Chapter One that everywhere in Still's writings are references to spirit, life, soul, and motion, all of which refer to the same force of vitalism. As we proceed to the next chapter and through the remainder of this book, this vitalistic principle is the central theme. Spirit is at the center of Still's philosophy. I intend to demonstrate for you that this elevated approach to medicine was indeed Still's orientation, and, if we choose to follow his lead today, we will re-create the practice of medicine to the liking of Osteopathy. The process to re-create it is already underway.

2

ELUCIDATING A. T. STILL

Form is the body of the spirit and is used by the spirit.
Without spirit, the form cannot move, and without form,
the spirit cannot exist.

— A. ELLIS, N. WISEMAN, AND K. BOSS[1]

In this chapter, we expand on the propositions of Andrew Taylor Still and compare them with other authors and paradigms. Chapter Two includes several layers of information. First, it investigates what those who personally knew Dr. Still said about him and his ideas. Then, it introduces thoughts similar to Still's from others who did not know him. It delves into the subject of Mind as Still enunciated it, and it looks at Mind's interaction with Matter. Then, this chapter addresses the common aspects of Still's philosophy with modern physics. Finally, it examines how Mind influences the practice of medicine and our lives in general.

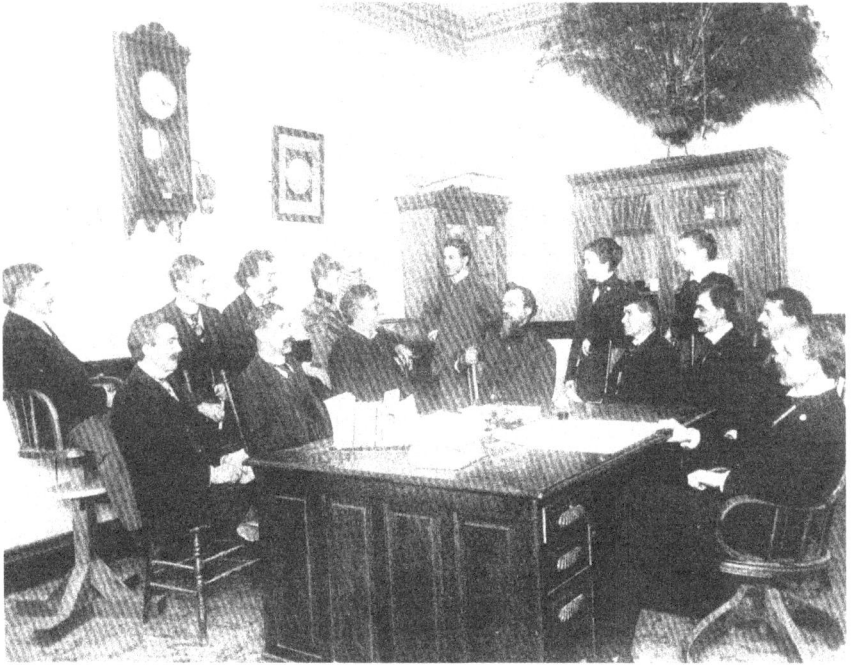

2.1 Faculty of the American School of Osteopathy, ca. 1898. (Reproduced from the *Journal of Osteopathy*, 1899.)

I. EARLY DEFINITION OF OSTEOPATHY

A. Associates of Still

From many sources,[2–7] we can discover the early thoughts of those who gathered around Still, learned from him, and developed the new profession. These people were the ones who had the first opportunity to infer what Andrew Still taught and practiced. Many of them interpreted Still's ideas using their own terms, just as we are doing now. They wanted to comprehend more clearly what Still wanted them to know in order to proceed more efficiently with the business of the new profession, especially looking toward the time when he would no longer be there to confer with. Booth described in his 1905 book, *History of Osteopathy* (394–397), various definitions of Osteopathy that emerged during the period while Still was living, when the profession was in the early stages of its development.

Booth mentioned a nephew of Mrs. A. T. Still, G. D. Hulett, DO, who, as professor of Osteopathic Practice in the early years of the American School of Osteopathy in Kirksville was one of the more authoritative individuals to comment on Still's philosophy. Hulett's 1903 book, *A Text Book of the Principles of Osteopathy,* considers the early formulation of the definition of Osteopathy by osteopaths other than Still:

> A technical definition must suggest a concept of the cause and the treatment of disease. In regard to the latter it must not only embrace therapeutics but prophylaxis as well. . . . In order that our definition shall include essentials and give to us a basis of support the following propositions must be either directly or by inference included:
>
> 1. Cure is the prerogative of the organism.
> 2. Functional disorders will be self-adjusted except where complicated with or dependent on structural disorders which are beyond the limits of self-adjustment.
> 3. Removal of structural disorders constitutes the treatment.

In accordance with these provisions we have in another publication (Journal of the American Osteopathic Association, May, 1902) (JAOA) suggested the following definition of osteopathy:

> "*A system of therapeutics which, recognizing that the maintenance and restoration of normal function are alike dependent on a force inherent in bioplasm, and that function perverted beyond the limits of self-adjustment, is dependent on a condition of structure perverted beyond those limits, attempts the re-establishment of normal function by manipulative measures designed to render the organism such aid as will enable it to overcome or adapt itself to the disturbed structure.*" (Hulett, 22)

B. Hulett's View of the Origins of Still's Concepts

1. Osteopathy Follows a Theory of Life

From G. D. Hulett's writings, we find similarities to the modern definition of Osteopathy: that healing comes from within the organism, that structure and function are related, and that addressing the structural disorder improves function and constitutes treatment. In contrast to the modern definition of Osteopathy, it is abundantly clear from the just-cited 1902 quotation from the *JAOA* that the young profession counted the life force as a fundamental precept of its philosophy. G. D. Hulett, DO, published his book when Still was still actively teaching in Kirksville. It is presumed that osteopathic treatises published at that time were reviewed by Still. Hulett stated, "A theory of life is at the basis of the osteopathic science" (12). Early in the osteopathic profession, the curriculum included the concept of the vital force within the protoplasm, as related to the structure-function interrelationship. The life force, or spirit, in the protoplasm was essential to the basis of the philosophy. Modern osteopathic curricula have deemphasized, if not eliminated, this fundamental concept.

2. Matter and Vitality

A second element in Hulett's definition that contrasts with modern osteopathic tenets was the inability at times of the structural component to self-adjust, while the functional component more readily self-adjusts. Hulett implied that, for protoplasm, no limitations are placed on function by form. However, once embryogenesis or development establishes a form for a specific, predetermined function, the form, if distorted, can interfere with the function. Perturbations of form interfere with function because material form cannot self-adjust as readily as function can. Material form derives from the Terrestrial Mother in Still's model, whereas function derives from the Celestial Father. The life force, or spirit, coming from the Celestial, must inject its influence in order for us to experience the Motion of life in the Terrestrial Matter. Without spirit, Matter remains relatively immobile, devitalized. I emphasize these three points: (1) the importance in osteopathic philosophy of the vital force in protoplasm, (2) the less vital character of the material substance of the body without the vital force, and (3) the consequent difficulty for the structural component to self-adjust as compared to the ease with which the functional component self-adjusts. These three points become critical in the development of a new model as this book unfolds.

3. Form and Function

To understand Hulett's interpretation of Still, let us read directly from his book.

> There is an organizing force that lies back of all structure. That force is unknown but it represents an action, an energy, a function. In this sense we are justified in insisting that function is a cause of structure. We may follow out this assertion, however, with the equally obvious statement that before that organizing force can express itself in any substantial way it must have a structural basis. That structural basis is protoplasm [biogen (for Still)]. In this view of the matter we are justified in claiming that structure governs function . . . In large part, it will be noted that the functioning energy only modifies the structure in the process of growth, compensation, or any condition where a definite purposeful action seems necessary . . . As soon as the functional activity . . . has builded [*sic*] its own instrument of manifestation, . . . thence on, . . . structure becomes modified only inappreciably and gradually by the function. The structure . . . is in considerable part unable to immediately adjust itself, with the result that the function must immediately suffer and continue so to do until the structural condition be overcome . . . Admitting that function can modify the structure, it much more readily can modify itself and hence is perfectly self-adjusting. On the other hand, structure is only passively self-adjustive, and hence

will likely remain in its abnormal condition until some external force is brought to bear . . . Structure representing the channels through which the life forces manifest themselves becomes comparatively unyielding. (Hulett, 26–27.)

Hulett summarized this line of thinking by saying, "All processes of healing are dependent on the inherent power of protoplasm; that that inherent power to heal will be exercised so long as structural conditions are normal" (63). We conclude from this that function, as a component from the spiritual realm, generates a material form that is less vital and requires the life force to move it. The material form must be moved by the life force or, once it becomes still, it declines toward death. Further, if the form is perturbed, some outside force is usually required to restore its original conformation and to permit the return of the life force, which is recognized as health. The process of the return of health to the tissues is healing.

4. Holism

Hulett cited, among others, Paracelsus (1493–1541) as having contributed to Dr. Still's concepts. Paracelsus said that (1) all nature is a unit; (2) nature is never complete but forever becoming; and (3) nature is a macrocosm, man a microcosm (Hulett, 14). Still's concept of "man" concurs with Paracelsus's. To paraphrase Still, the body is a hieroglyphical representation of worlds.[8]

There are many demonstrations of holism in our world. The holograph (mathematically theorized in 1947 by Dennis Gabor, for which he later received the Nobel Prize) helps explain, in modern scientific terms, the concept of holism. To produce a holograph of a particular object—first accomplished in 1965 by Emmett Leith and Juris Upatnicks as lasers became available—we split a laser beam (coherent light) into two, one reflecting off the object and the other, the reference beam, converging slightly out of phase onto a medium to develop the image. If the image is developed onto a glass plate, what appears on the glass, because the two laser beams are out of phase, is a disorganized array of shimmering colors, representing an interference pattern. However, when illuminated with a laser, this interference pattern on the glass plate casts into mid-air a three-dimensional ghostly image of the object. If the glass plate is shattered, each fragment, when illuminated, will cast a similar image of the whole object, with its intensity and clarity diminished proportionately according to the size of the fragment relative to the whole plate of glass. Thus, each part represents the whole. The holographic image exists without material substance, but represents the material substance. Although it is a photographic process, holography is unique in that the image appears in space and each part casts an image of the whole.[9] Still asserted that the human form is cast of material earthly elements from an image provided by the Celestial realm of spirit and that the body represents a microcosm of the cosmos. Rupert Sheldrake described a mechanism by which patterns of energy lay out the blueprint for the structural conformation of each organism. (See Section II.D: "Rupert Sheldrake").

5. Healing Generates from Within

According to Still:

It appears perfectly reasonable to any person born above the condition of an idiot, who has familiarized himself with anatomy and its working with the machinery of life, that all diseases are mere effects, the cause being a partial or complete failure of the nerves to properly conduct the fluids of life.[10]

Hulett also pointed to Thomas Sydenham, the seventeenth-century English physician, as an influence on Still's thinking. Sydenham contended that healing comes from nature. In the early 1800s, Krukenberg expanded Sydenham's view and said, "Physicians should be filled with a pious reverence toward nature; the organism is a whole and must be contemplated in this sense; medical art is undoubtedly capable of decisive action, but let us not mistake that in many cases its activity is quite superfluous, in very many null and inadequate, and in many injurious" (in Hulett, 17). Of course, a major premise of A. T. Still was that the organism furnishes all the necessary substances for its own health to produce healing from within. He honored nature, and at the same time he condemned the drugs of his day for their injurious effects and decried the medical profession for its ignorance about the drugs it used and its other ineffective methods. Oliver Wendell Holmes, Sr., MD, declared in 1860, "If the whole *materia medica* as now used could be sunk to the bottom of the sea, it would be all the better for mankind—and all the worse for the fishes."[11]

6. Biogen: The First Product of Life

Hulett indicated that Still proclaimed living tissue (biogen, bioplasm, or protoplasm), not the cell, to be the first product of the life essence. Although Hulett acknowledged Virchow's recently declared cell doctrine, that the cell is the basic unit of life, he reiterated that Still disagreed, believing that spirit's first evidence of material manifestation was biogen. Biogen is pluripotent, living tissue that has not yet become specialized. It is protoplasm, the simplest example of Matter in Motion.

In accordance with this view is the work of a modern German physician, Alfred Pischinger, MD.[12] Pischinger included the connective tissue matrix and nutrient capillary along with the cell as the basic functional unit of life. He has "taken the cell isolated by Virchow out of its abstraction and placed it in the triad of the capillary, the basic [ground] substance, and the cell, as the smallest common functional denominator of life in a vertebrate organism" (Pischinger, 18). We return to Pischinger's ideas in the next chapters.

7. Moving Equilibrium

> The most striking characteristic of living tissue is its tendency to con-
> tinual change . . . and since life may be considered in large part a response
> to stimuli the necessity for the ability to change becomes apparent . . .
> In the sense of a continuous response to continuous stimuli the organ-
> ism constitutes a *moving equilibrium.* When that equilibrium becomes
> disturbed by too intense or too prolonged stimuli disease results, while
> in the continuous adjustment to circumstances we have the normal
> condition of the living organism maintained. (Hulett, 24–25)

In the mid- and late 1800s in Germany, Traube, Hering, and Mayer discovered a moving equilibrium in the average arterial pressure of dogs. The pulse pressure, systole minus diastole, remained about the same, but the average pressure of the blood in the vessel varied with a cycle occur- ring at a rate of approximately six times a minute. Mayer discovered a longer wave, about two times a minute. The author of physiology texts, Arthur C. Guyton, MD, studied these oscillations of blood pressure and found the variability to be independent from respiratory activity. He speculated that the oscillation represents a searching about a mean pressure, which is under neuronal control. We come back to the idea of a moving equilibrium in succeeding chapters.

II. OTHER AUTHORS AND PARADIGMS

A. Emmanuel Swedenborg—Spirit Invests Itself With Matter

The writings of Emmanuel Swedenborg might have influenced Drew Still. We know that Still was involved with the local community of Swedenborgians who were Spiritualists, many of whom emigrated from the source of Spiritualism in New York State to Lawrence, Kansas, in the late1850s in order to assure that Kansas would be admitted to the Union as a free state.[13] Dr. Still is quoted in Booth's 1905 *History of Osteopathy* as saying that the evidence that the Spiritualists produced through séances "consoled" him (see Chapter Two, Section VI). These spiritual exercises proved to Still that the human spirit persists after death and that earthly life, in the ongoing existence of the spirit, is a special case in which spirit invests itself with a physical form. This conclusion by Still is evident in much of his writing (see Chapter One).

Swedenborg, an anatomist, physiologist, Christian mystic, and philosopher, developed his ideas in Sweden from 1688 to 1772. From his experiments with live dogs and dissections of many human cadavers, Swedenborg compiled several volumes on medical subjects, including *The Brain*[14-15] and *The Cerebrum*.[16-17] He is credited with being the first to record, in 1736, the independent respiratory activity of the brain and the circulatory and pulsatile activity of the cerebrospinal fluid (Swedenborg 1882, xvi).

In his smallest work, *De Commercio Animae et Corporis* (1769), translated as *Intercourse of the Soul and the Body*, Swedenborg declared that he was an authority on matters of the spirit as well as the body because he was privileged by God to have been exposed to both the spiritual and the physical realms while living. He asserted that he knew the truth of the interrelation of the soul and the body because he had witnessed it firsthand.[18-19] He affirmed that he had been shown that from God comes a spiritual influx and "clothes itself with that which is natural, as a man clothes himself with a garment." Like Still, Swedenborg indicated that wisdom (Mind, for Still) derives from the realm of spirit and that the action of the body (Motion, for Still) is a further effect from this same source, the love of God (Swedenborg 1769, x). Still believed, as did Swedenborg, that the motion of the body derives from the Celestial life or spirit. Perhaps both men developed their models independently; although the construction of their models is similar, their terms are different. Of course, Swedenborg wrote in Latin, offering various options for translation.

1. Soul Creates Form

There are no causes in the observable world . . . The observable world is a world of effects. — DAVID HAWKINS

Swedenborg went on to say, "Spiritual things, thus clothed in a man, enabled him to live as a rational and moral man, thus as a spiritually natural man" (1769, 1). He said, "The soul is properly the universal essence of its body" (Swedenborg 1882, 64). "For what can truly be, unless it be from a thing prior, more simple, and more unique, which is the beginning of the rest? That which gives to others being and existence, must itself be. The soul also is peculiar [individualized] and proper [suitable and compatible], and there is not one universal soul for all; so that the soul of one cannot belong to the body of another; for, what is to be demonstrated, namely, the very *form* of the body is the result of its essential [spiritual] determination, or the body itself represents the soul as it were in an *image*" (Swedenborg 1882, 64; italics added).

2. Spirit Invests Itself with Matter

Still characterized this spiritual influence on the physical form as a "substance."

> (1) Life surely is a very finely prepared *substance,* which is the all-moving force of Nature, or that force that moves all nature from worlds to atoms. It seems to be a *substance* that contains all the principles of construction [form] and motion [function], with the power to endow that which it constructs with the attributes necessary to the object it has formulated from matter and sent forth as a living being. We think it is not unreasonable to conclude that life is matter in motion. (Still 1892, 256–257; italics added)

Still's description of the process of vivifying the human form with the "all-moving force of Nature" was similar to the model (see Fig. 2.2)

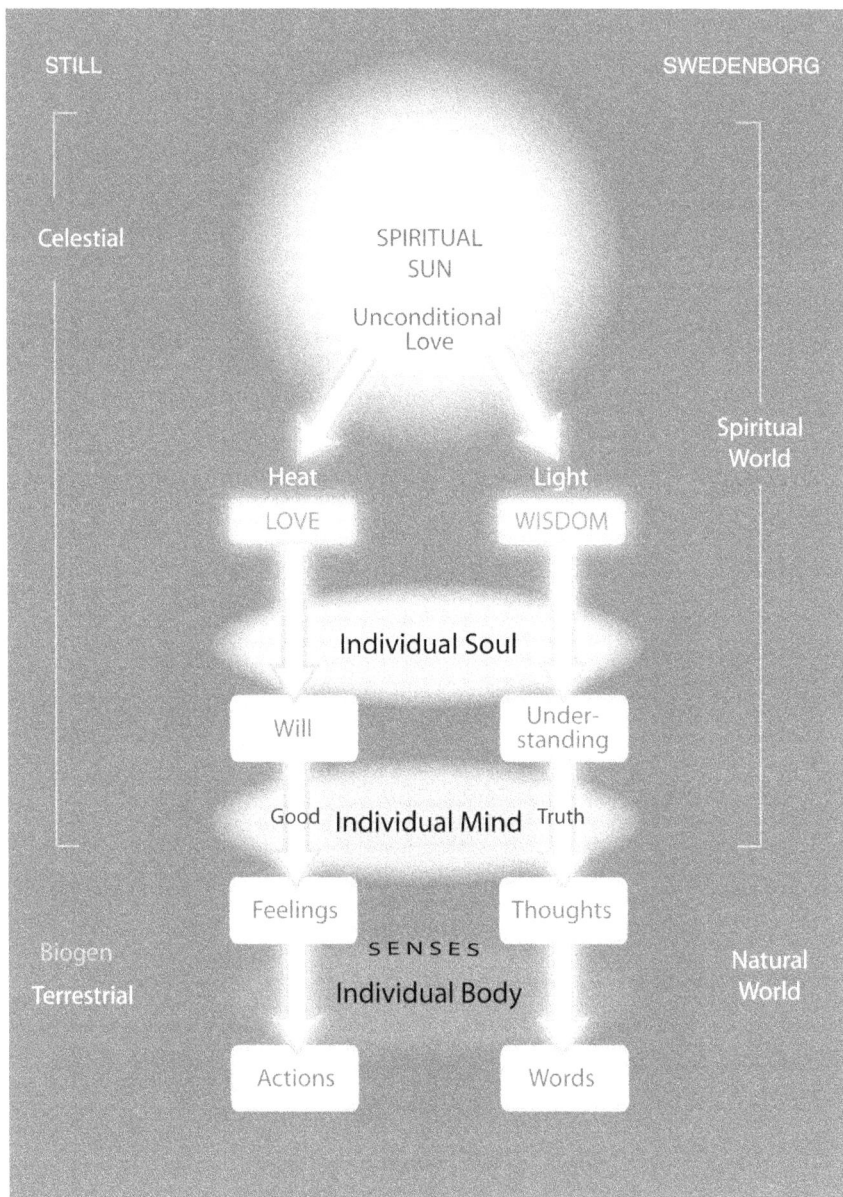

2.2   Diagram of Emmanuel Swedenborg's philosophy produced from his *Intercourse of the Soul and Body* (1769) republished 1947 London: The Swedenborg Society. Radiation in the form of heat and light emanating from the spiritual sun clothes itself with a physical form and creates human attributes of will, understanding, feelings, thoughts, speech, and action. The diagram also shows a comparison of Still's philosophy opposite Swedenborg's. Original art by Raychel Ciemma.

from Emmanuel Swedenborg (1769, 1–61), who said, "That which is spiritual clothes itself with that which is natural [material], as a man clothes himself with a garment." Swedenborg also described how spirit emanates from God and flows into the soul of man. He described where this vitalizing force could be discovered in the body when he said, "Life is found in the juices between the fibers." Swedenborg differentiated the inactive Terrestrial from the vital Celestial. "The lower essences have derived from the inert and heavier elements of the world this feature, that they are able to coalesce into a lower essence, and to be of use to functions in the ultimate parts of the world" (Swedenborg 1882, 66).

To summarize, Swedenborg indicated in these writings that the soul creates the human form from less active earthly material and then clothes itself in this material form, vitalizing it. Hulett's writing drew similar conclusions. If we compare Still's quotations in Chapter One with Swedenborg's ideas, we see a remarkable similarity between the models of these two philosophers (see Sections II.A.5 and 6: "Human Is Triune" and "Form and Motion"). Still also said:

(2) The mind is asked to find the connection between the physical and the spiritual . . . Life . . . must have definite arrangements by which it can be united and act with matter. (Still 1892, 249)

In this quotation, Still entertained the manner by which spirit invests itself with matter, just as Swedenborg described. The interaction of the two, spirit and Matter, creates form and Motion, the two requirements of life. This interaction, according to Still involves a reciprocal activity between the Celestial and the Terrestrial realms.

In a similar respect, Danté said, "The Love of God, unutterable and perfect, flows into a pure soul the way that light rushes into a transparent object." This image of a substance flowing from God into humans is similar to the models expressed by Swedenborg and Still. The image created by these three men, Danté, Swedenborg, and Still is one of a sea of energy (the love of God) from which the living form is created, in which it continues to exist, and by which it is nourished.

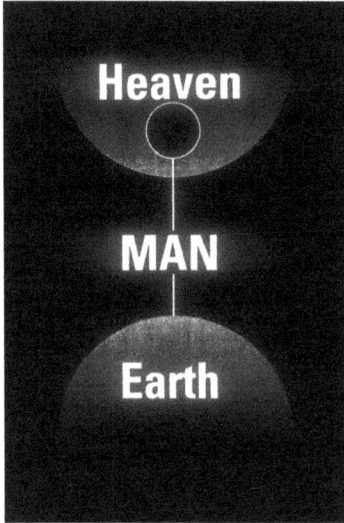

2.3 Diagram showing the relationships of heaven, earth, and man in traditional Chinese philosophy. Arms extending towards heaven demarcate the celestial orb while descending legs delineate the earthly orb. Original art by Brian Epp.

B. Traditional Chinese Medicine—*Qi*

Qi (or *Chi*) is the mover in Traditional Chinese Medicine (TCM). TCM characterizes reality in a way similar to Still. In this cultural belief system, it is said that Heaven (Celestial Father, for Still) fecundates Earth (Terrestrial Mother, for Still) to create Life (form and Motion, for Still).[20] According to the Taoist Chinese, this activity of fecundation to create life traces the movement of *Qi*.[21] A limited English translation of "*Qi*" is energy or vital force. If we think of *Qi* as equivalent to vital force (life force) for the purposes of this book, we can make a direct comparison of the Chinese philosophy with Still's. Summarizing this comparison, we can say the vital force activates and nourishes the material substance to produce a life form in motion. (Lee, 32–33) This summary compares favorably with our discussion of Swedenborg as well.

Still said:

(4) **Life surely is a very finely prepared substance, which is the all-moving force of Nature, or that force that moves all nature from worlds to atoms.** (Still 1892, 256)

In this statement, Still described what the Chinese believe are the activities of *Qi*. *Qi* in China, *ki* in Japan, and *prana* in India, are three terms used by three cultures out of many, that identify a vitalistic principle. All three cultures indicate that this element of nature activates and nourishes all matter. Any motion, from Brownian movement and the principles of thermodynamics, to chemistry and physiological activities, to gross motions of wind and volcanoes, and to human activities of speech and dance, derives its movement from *Qi*.

The conceptual concurrence of *Qi* (Chinese) and life (Still), which both activate matter, makes us wonder whether Still borrowed his ideas from the Chinese. However, no author who wrote about Still ever referred to Chinese thought as an influence on his thinking, nor did Still

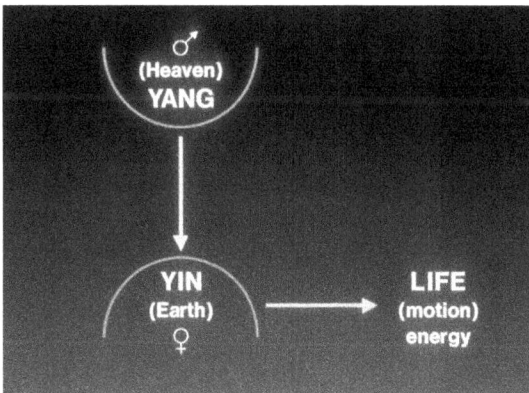

2.4 This diagram depicts the movement of Qi in which yang fecundates yin and produces life according to traditional Chinese philosophy. Original art by Brian Epp.

himself. Whatever the influence on Still, he was clearly an independent thinker in his own right as he testified in the first statement of one of his books, "I quote no authors but God and experience" (Still 1892, 9). It is clear that both philosophies merely use different words to describe the same basic truth of nature.

C. Native Americans—No-Form into Form

Like the Chinese and other traditional societies whose cultures emerged as one continuous stream from prehistory into the present, the Native Americans also held similar perspectives about the natural order. But, in this case, it is highly likely that the Shawnee Indians influenced Still. He lived and worked with these people as he "read medicine" (precepted) under his father, Abram. In these formative years of 1853 and 1854, Andrew, then 25 years old, lived with his wife, two children, his parents, and the transplanted Shawnee Indians in an isolated encampment that they constructed twenty-five miles west of Kansas City and two miles off the trail leading to California. Once the Kansas-Nebraska Bill was passed in 1854, the first homesteaders entered the region. But until then, no other white people were allowed into Kansas because it was legally Indian Territory. Communication at the Wakarusa mission, outside of the English-speaking school, was in the Shawnee language (Still 1908, 56). The Stills became close friends with Paschal Fish, the chief of the Shawnee band that Fish had brought to Kansas from Ohio. The Indians had been displaced, as were the Stills who had come from Missouri to this new and undeveloped place where they all had to make a new life together. No doubt, a community developed out of necessity, although Martha, Andrew's mother, felt shear loneliness and grief most of the time. She was forced to relive, moment by moment, her childhood trauma and grief from having watched most of her family killed by this very same band of Shawnee Indians decades earlier in Ohio (Trowbridge, 38–46).

As Andrew began to "doctor" patients, to share food and community, he said, "I soon learned to speak their tongue" (Still 1908, 57). With language comes an understanding of a cultural view of reality, and Still demonstrated his affinity for their culture by using their language. In his *Autobiography*, Still wrote in Shawnee, "Illnoywa Tapamala-qua," which signifies the life and mind of the living God (1908, 241). In a speech given at the fiftieth anniversary of the survivors of the members of the Kansas Free-State Legislature in 1907, Still was asked by the governor of Kansas what year he had arrived in the state, to which Still replied, "1853." Surprised, the governor sarcastically responded by saying that he must have lived with the Indians, because there were no white people in the state yet. Still, then 79 years old, stood waving his cane and reeled off a string of words in Shawnee to prove that he had indeed lived with the Indians.[22]

What could Still have learned from his close association with the Native Americans? Primary to traditional peoples, the Taoist Chinese and American Indians alike, is the notion of vitality in everything. The Chinese have given it a name, *Qi*. Among Native Americans, there frequently are no names provided, only actions. Most Indian words describe vital behaviors, even words that are translated into English as nouns. All is seen as active and alive, even things that our western culture thinks of as inanimate. Spirit is in everything. From Joseph Rael comes this insight about perceiving reality as alive: "My life as a half-breed living among the Utes, then the Picuris pueblans and then the whites, has taught me the difference between mental perceptions and vibrational perceptions. With a mental perception, the human psyche first creates movement and quickly gives it placement, defines it; whereas, a vibrational perception, or intuition, comes as an awareness of a vibration carrying the essence of the thing perceived. Definition (placement) is not necessary for vibrational perception. It comes with a resonance, grounded in an awareness of its own inner alive knowing. It comes complete, like a flower, or a song. Instantly we perceive it in its fullness; we drink its light and it becomes part of us."[23]

This type of perception is common to traditional peoples of the world. The Chinese written language is ideographic, each character representing an idea or action complete and full, with nuances and shades of meaning, history, and richness of associations all available at once in a glance, not linear and sterile, as is this string of words on this page. Instead of stringing letters, words, sentences, and paragraphs together to make some sense out of images, the Chinese communicate images. So too, the Chinese think holographically, just as Joseph Rael describes the functioning of his Native American thinking and language. This is the manner by which dolphins communicate, in many frequencies of sounds, all at once, to transmit an image of a swimmer thrashing in the water, afraid, heavy wet clothes impairing his movement, blowing bubbles, and drowning; and, at the same time, "Let's lift him gently and quickly to the surface for air." Instead, using this language as expressed on this page with its accompanying paradigm, we must dictate this picture linearly, wasting time in doing so; and the swimmer may not be saved. Our linear thinking and mode of expression leave us far behind in comprehending a holographic universe. Dr. Still thought, talked, and wrote holographically, despite the handicap of having to use linear English.

Naming a thing ("placement" in Rael's terms) threatens the one who names it with getting stuck in form. "Forms lead us toward attachments, and attachments glue us to a set time and place, hence suffering. Picuris people don't call themselves Picuris. They call themselves *tuu taah teh nay* and then *pii-tah*—where the center of life is, or where the kiva* is

---

* The *kiva* is the center of the life of the puebloan peoples. It is a covered, circular depression in their pueblo structures (ancient and modern) in which they hold ceremonies recognizing their ancestors and origins. They believe they originate as spirit within the earth from which they emerge into physical existence through the *sipapu*, a small, dark hole in the center of the floor of the *kiva*. Light is supplied by a fire next to the *sipapu* and through the roof, which is covered by branches. Thus, we see the dark and light of nonexistence and existence, respectively.

the center. 'We are the people from the source—the center of the circle of light.'. . . They're calling themselves 'the No-form creating the form.' This is what they represent. It's what they are . . . *tuu taah teh nay* . . . suggests that they don't exist, but that also suggests that they do exist in states of non-existence. Non-existence is what gives validity to existence. Non-existence is black, and existence is white" (Rael, 46). (Section II.H, about David Bohm and Section II.I, about William Tiller, have more on the dichotomy between nonexistence and existence.)

Spiritual presence is also central to Dr. Still's philosophy—and to this book. Whether he actually received it from the Native Americans or derived it spontaneously from his own unique experience, Still nevertheless had a ready source for the idea of a holographic universe and spiritual embodiment in material reality through his close and undisturbed encounter with the Shawnee Indians during a two-year "preceptorship" on the lonely Kansas prairie. The notion of spiritual embodiment is consistent with concepts from Swedenborg as well.

Lori Arviso Alvord, MD, a Navajo surgeon graphically depicted the disparity of approach between conventional and traditional forms of viewing reality.[24] She described the contradiction between the two worldviews of the Navajo medicine man and the Centers for Disease Control and Prevention (CDC) in the case of the Hantavirus. When one of Alvord's patients succumbed to the then unknown disease in 1993, a Navajo medicine man (*hataalii)* was consulted and he indicated, "The illness was caused by too much rainfall, which had caused the piñon trees to bear too much fruit. The unexpectedly large harvest of piñon nuts was a significant deviation from the natural harmony of the world . . . this was what was causing the people to become sick. While the epidemiologists were looking for the solution in their microscopes, the *hataalii* had looked to the macro level—disturbed natural patterns in the universe" (Alvord, 120–121).

The *hataalii* revealed photographs of sand paintings used in healing ceremonies for this illness by medicine men decades earlier, which contained the image of a tiny mouse in the lower corner of the sand painting. The large harvest of piñon nuts had increased the population of mice. The *hataalii* said to the CDC investigators, "Look to the mouse." At the CDC, a virus contracted from the droppings of the deer mouse was eventually isolated and determined to be the cause. Guidance from the *hataalii* directed the search at the CDC, yet nowhere was credit for this imparted information from the Navajo healers reported in the press. Despite the disparity of the two worldviews and the two healing approaches, when integrated they could provide a greater whole from which the health of the people benefited.

D. Rupert Sheldrake—Morphic Fields

Rupert Sheldrake, in his book *A New Science of Life*,[25] first theorized the concept of morphogenetic fields to explain how plants create form while growing and developing. He indicated that all living things follow a generalized, established pattern (morphic field) to create each unique individual organism. These patterns exist beyond biochemistry, genetics, and our normal set of expectations. Morphic fields exist as imprints of information or consciousness outside physical reality, memorized from previous material forms, from which each new physical form takes its cue. Sheldrake described "modified materialism," affirming the reality that all material substance is basically energy (Sheldrake 1981, 200). Many other authors agree.[26–28]

In summary, Sheldrake acknowledged an unseen world of consciousness or information (Mind, for Still) that serves as an organizing principle for the world of material reality ("forms wisely constructed," for Still). This world of consciousness (Celestial Father, for Still) patterns the world of material substance (Terrestrial Mother, for Still) to engender a living form (man, for Still).

(3) Thus, we have the union of mind, matter, and life.
(Still 1892, 251–252)

Thus, Still and Sheldrake agreed that physical forms that contain life generate from unseen informational patterns. The hologram and Mandelbrot's mathematics can help us visualize this process.

E. Benoit Mandelbrot—Fractal Geometry

As a mathematician, Mandelbrot wanted to quantify the measurement of a seacoast, a pattern of stars in the sky, and the conformation of a mountain ridge. In the process of developing his mathematics, he eventually coined the term "fractal." A fractal refers to a demonstration within higher mathematics of shapes whose dimensionality is not a whole number, that is, a fraction. These shapes are irregular. "Since algebra derives from the Arabic *jabara* = to bind together, *fractal* and *algebra* are etymological opposites."[29] The words "open-ended" and "infinite" thus describe fractal geometry. Through fractal geometry, Mandelbrot delved into the field of chaos. "Many scholars question the use of randomness in science; now the hope has arisen that it will be justified via fractal attractors" (Mandelbrot, 193). The term "attractor" in chaos theory refers to the attraction of mathematical sets of numbers to a point, a near circle, or other Euclidian shapes. In nonlinear dynamical systems, such as in nature, however, Mandelbrot contended that almost none of the attractors are shapes from Euclid; rather, they are fractals, irregular and disconnected. Further, studying fractals elucidates randomness, according to Mandelbrot. Thus, chaos theory and fractal geometry have much in common.

Fractals demonstrate another characteristic of nature: iterations of form through changes of scale. An example of this is the similarity of form among the branches on a tree, the twigs on the branches, and the veins in the leaves. Another example is the iterations of form demonstrated by solar systems and atoms. Iterations of form also occur across phyla in the animal kingdom. For example, the ratio 1 : 2 : 5 represents the bones in the extremities, which manifest in the human body as humerus (1), radius and ulna (2), and the metacarpals and digits (5). One of Mandelbrot's conclusions about his mathematics was that it describes forms that develop from forces of nature. Thus, in Mandelbrot's work we see the evidence in higher mathematics for the manner in which forms spontaneously take shape in nature. Further, his fractal geometry describes holography; that is, minute areas of a form appear symmetrical to and reiterate the whole (Mandelbrot, 468).

Mandelbrot used mathematics to show that the amorphous complexity of nature has patterns that can be elucidated and described. His "geometry of nature" described things that we can see and feel. For the first time, mathematics, a tool of science, elucidated for us experiences of the first order instead of creating models (of the second order) to examine natural phenomena. Such artificial models separate us from nature and ourselves. Mandelbrot's geometry lets us see manifestations of flow, form, and vitality that occur in nature. This math connects science and art, nature with philosophy, and ourselves to ourselves. Fractal geometry offers us a mathematical means to confirm Sheldrake's morphic fields, natural conformations of energy that determine the shape of material bodies.

F. Max Planck—Quantum Mechanics

In 1900, Max Planck, a physicist, introduced to the world the idea of quanta—tiny discrete bundles of energy that behave both like a wave and a particle. This formed the basis of quantum physics. Here are the basic premises of quantum physics:

1. A quantum object (for example, an electron) can be at more than one place at a time.

2. A quantum object cannot be said to manifest in ordinary space-time until we observe it as a particle.

3. When a quantum object ceases to exist here and simultaneously appears in existence over there, we cannot say it went through the intervening space (the quantum leap).

4. A manifestation of one quantum object, caused by our observation, simultaneously influences its correlated twin object—no matter how far apart they are (quantum action at a distance; nonlocality).

These concepts are still percolating through our consciousness and have begun to deeply affect many aspects of our perception of reality. Lasers, transistors, and computerized axial tomography (CAT) scans all are evidence of a shift in our thinking and the consequent production of devices that enhance our lives. Nevertheless, our day-to-day existence still has not caught up with what quantum physics tells us about the true nature of our reality. Concepts in medicine, for example, continue to lag behind. In fact, scientific medicine operates from a perspective that comes from the Cartesian split of mind and body and Newtonian cause-and-effect mechanical physics from the seventeenth century.

What would medicine look like if it integrated the ideas of modern physics? Simply put, it would look osteopathic. The rest of this book explores what this means. Still comprehended the effects of nonlocality as a Spiritualist. Still understood the unity of everything. He taught that the body was vivified by spirit, a hieroglyphical representation of All-That-Is. He recognized the primary role of Mind in creation and in the function of the human organism. He projected that the mind could do what an x-ray machine does, that is, raise the vibration to see inside a material body.

G. Larry Dossey—Eternity Medicine

In his book *Reinventing Medicine*,[30] Larry Dossey, MD, described three eras of medicine. Era I is characterized by a conventional, cause-and-effect, statistical, scientific approach to healing dating from the seventeenth century. It was responsible for the achievements in public health, clean water, and sewer systems, the eradication or control of communicable diseases, the development of antibiotics, trauma teams, and heroic heart surgery. Era II medicine is mind-body medicine. Here, medicine's most recent advances include psychosomatic and various alternative medical techniques, such as yoga, meditation, biofeedback, and the study of the nature of the placebo effect. Yet Dossey pointed out that the methods used to evaluate or study these Era II methods still resort to the same causal, statistical, deterministic proofs of Era I medicine. These Era I methods label mind-body phenomena "psycho-somatics" and "placebo response," trying to explain mind-body healing through physiology. In other words, there still has not been a shift of paradigm.

Dossey predicted that the shift of paradigm will occur with Era III medicine—this is nonlocal medicine or eternity medicine. Here, the mind plays a fundamental role in the healing of the patient. This form of medicine integrates the concepts of quantum physics. Intention plays a significant role in healing, both from the mind of the physician and the mind of the patient. However, this type of medicine cannot be measured by conventional means. As Denney, a modern philosopher, put it: "Paradoxically, that imposed science by its very nature cannot measure the nonlinear, subjective, whole, qualitative, open-ended, and spiritual ways of the quantum leaps of nonlocal, soul-body healing."[31]

Within Dossey's model is something very reminiscent of the concept of Mind, Matter, and Motion that Still proclaimed over a century ago. Returning to these formative concepts of osteopathic medicine puts the spirit back into the principles and practice. As Dossey proclaimed,

"People everywhere are starved for meaning, purpose, and spiritual fulfillment in their lives"(11). Still's earnest thirsting for knowledge about the nature of life and spirit drove him to the discovery of Osteopathy (see Section IV: "Still's Clairvoyance and Spiritualism"). His experience with Spiritualism and his dreams and visions that are documented in his *Autobiography* demonstrate to us today how much Still was involved with the aspect of Mind (consciousness) in his everyday life. His life is an example for us, a means by which we can bridge the gulf between Era II and Era III medicines. This reach for spiritual meaning plays out in our search for health and healing.

Denney wrote: "Instead of trying to measure quanta with an old science, we might open-mindedly enter into mysteries, thereby allowing our inquiry to include subjectivity, quality, open-ended discovery, and spirit. Once we enter this poetic and imaginative realm of soul-body healing, we can make a quantum shift not only in consciousness but in paradigm" (22).

Rael pointed out, "Maybe we have gotten too caught up in technology and now is the time that technology has reached its highest potential. Now it's time for us to reawaken and move to the total opposite of technology where we rely on the supernatural powers that were here before we came to inhabit the earth. So, if I want to fly across a railroad early in the morning like I once saw a Navajo medicine man do, or if I want to have telescopic sight, or if I want to be able to disappear and reappear in another place randomly, now is the time. Over time everything becomes its opposite. Now is the time for the opposite to happen. That way technology can be complemented by the No-form" (153).

H. David Bohm—Implicate and Explicate Orders

A physicist and colleague of Albert Einstein, David Bohm theorized that the universe is a hologram. He concluded that two realities exist simultaneously, one that we routinely experience and the other more subtle and hidden that underlies the first. The former he called the "explicate order," the latter, the "implicate order." The implicate, or enfolded (more subtle and hidden), order is mother and father to the explicate, or unfolded, order (everyday reality). What appears to be stable and tangible in the visible world of the explicate order is not truly there but emerges through a process of holomovement from a more primary and invisible implicate order of the universe. The implicate order includes the explicate order. Or, to put it another way, the explicate order is a part of the whole, which is the implicate order. The relationship between the explicate and implicate orders demonstrates a principle of holographic reality. Like the cloud in the air, the "material substance" (cloud) is created and moved by and within the inclusive "unmanifest" (air). In this analogy, the cloud represents the explicate order, and the air, the implicate order. Although air is composed of matter, it is used to represent the unseen implicate order. Actually, Bohm indicated that the implicate order is indeed composed of a subtle form of matter, which is consciousness.

In fact, the explicate order is purely vibration, as is the implicate order. Solid matter is not solid at all. Instead, it is basically vibration. We experience objects as being solid because the negative charges of the electrons vibrating in the object and in our hands, repel each other. Essentially, there is no stable substance to identify other than the vibrations of atoms. But there is more "empty" space between the nucleus and orbiting electrons than there is substance. The substances of the atoms are defined as probabilities, not definite elements in a particular place at a particular time. Subatomic particles that make up the atoms emerge from an undifferentiated background and then wink off again to be replaced by another appearance of vibration. This is the fundamental act of manifestation of our material reality, holomovement. "Holomovement" is the name Bohm gave the process by which the explicate order emerges from the implicate order. Holomovement is the emergence of matter from a preexisting pattern of energy. Such a pattern of energy compares to Sheldrake's concept of morphogenetic field.

According to Bohm, consciousness exists within both the unmanifest implicate order and the manifest explicate order. Consciousness contains thought, will, and emotion—the entire mental and emotional life. Bohm described consciousness as a subtler aspect of matter and movement. Consciousness is a subtle aspect of holomovement. It is what underlies matter and what moves it. Bohm said that consciousness or "nonmanifest matter is playing a role similar to what we thought of as *spirit*" (in Wilber, 65; italics added).

Bohm indicated that each living organism emerges out of a nonmanifest energy. According to Bohm, we can understand whether a living organism is diseased or healthy only through its nonmanifest aspect. When we treat a living entity, we consider the whole unseen movement: its nutrition, its light, and its chemistry.

To summarize Bohm's theory of a holistic universe, we can say that material reality (explicate order) emerges from an undifferentiated, unseen sea of consciousness (implicate order), which itself is a subtle form of matter. Consciousness (Mind, for Still) creates the material form (Matter, for Still) and moves it (Motion, for Still). So, Still's aspect of Mind is continuous throughout Bohm's model. That is, consciousness makes up the hidden and real worlds, creates the pattern for the unfoldment of material reality, and then moves it. For Bohm, consciousness is found to exist and to act in all of Still's elements of Mind, Matter, and Motion. Bohm said that in his model consciousness behaves in ways that we have attributed to spirit. It also behaves in ways that the Taoists have attributed to *Qi*.

Still's statements about life concur not only with the Taoists, but also with David Bohm. Still depicted life to be a substance,[32] and Bohm conceived consciousness to be a form of subtle matter found in the implicate order and acting to move the explicate order. Thus, we may infer that life (according to Still), *Qi* (according to the Taoists), and consciousness (according to Bohm) can be considered the same.

I. William Tiller—Particulate and Wave Spaces

William Tiller, PhD,[33–34] professor emeritus of the Department of Materials Science, Stanford University, studied the nature of consciousness and its effects on inanimate objects for several decades. His profound conclusions herald a new interpretation of reality by scientists, one that A. T. Still predicted 125 years ago with his philosophy based on Mind, Matter, and Motion. Tiller indicated that his model of physical reality is compatible with David Bohm's,[35] adding to Bohm's concepts a mathematical elucidation.

Tiller defined two worlds: one, a coarse particulate space, and the other, an information wave space. These two spaces are reciprocals of each other. They are derived from thermodynamics involving mathematical singularities plus de Broglie's concept of a particle and its pilot wave. The coarse particulate reality is governed by Maxwell's equations of electromagnetism, which are accepted by most physicists as the single representation of the physical universe. The information wave reality, proposed by Tiller as a logical extension of de Broglie's original proposition, doubles the dimensions of the universe as defined by Maxwell's equations.

Tiller had realized that we do not experience magnetic monopoles in our everyday reality. Only in theoretic nuclear realms, defined by quantum physics, and in other states of reality that we do not ordinarily experience do we find magnetic monopoles coexisting with electric monopoles. Tiller believed this demanded a mathematical explanation. Consequently, he created an outer and inner duplex reference frame for observations of nature, thereby unifying the nonordinary and ordinary aspects of physical space. This extended Maxwell's electromagnetic definitions into magnetoelectric realms.

In creating the reciprocal of Maxwell's equations, Tiller actually defined "etheric matter" in mathematical terms. By these new equations, Tiller also found a mathematical means for describing human aspects that until then had evaded scrutiny by scientists. He studied these human aspects of consciousness, mind, emotions, intention, and spirit, as related to their effects on water (change of pH), enzyme systems (behavior of alkaline phosphatase), and the rate of development of fruit fly larvae (based on the change of the ratio of ATP/ADP). He proved that devices programmed by human intention can robustly affect the three systems that he evaluated.

In his experiments, people with great experience in meditation programmed an electronic device that he invented. They programmed the device with a particular intention, for example, to elevate the pH of water by 1 pH unit. A similar electronic device to be used as a control

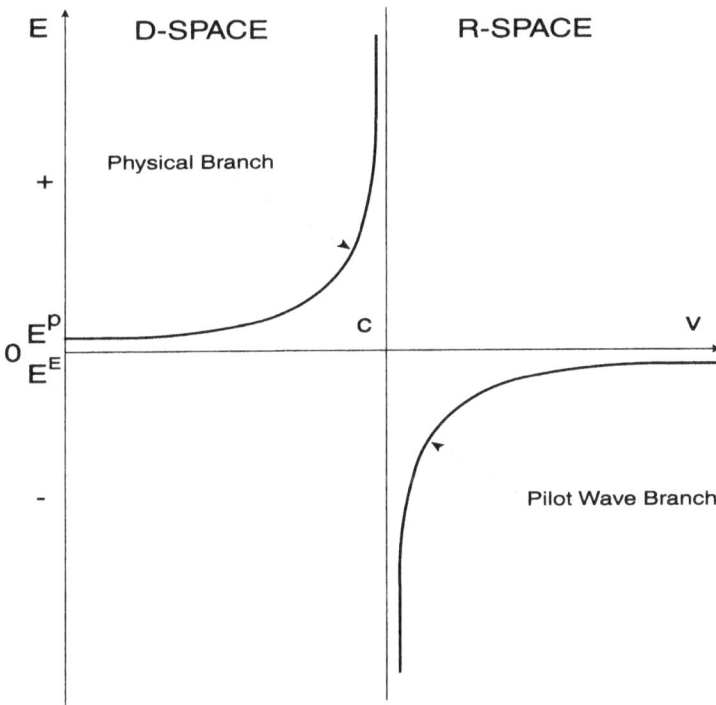

2.5   Mathematics of Tiller. This graph shows that by inverting mathematical equations that are fundamental to present day physics, our view of reality is greatly expanded. D-Space particles are those traveling at less than the speed of light while R-Space waves are those traveling at twice the speed of light. Through the delineation of R-Space, Tiller has theoretically and practically opened our horizons to include in scientific considerations the heretofore unincorporated factors of mind, emotion, and spirit. (Reproduced with permission from Tiller WA, Dibble WE, and Kohane MJ (2001). *Conscious Acts of Creation.* Walnut Creek, CA: Pavior Publishing. Fig 8.7, p. 331.)

was placed in metal foil in a Faraday cage, insulating it from electro-magnetic influences, next to the device being charged by the group of meditators. Later, these electronic devices were placed near a container of water. Measurements of the pH revealed a gradual but persistent movement of the hydrogen ion concentration in the direction of the intention until the intended level was achieved. The intention to lower the pH of the same type of purified water by one unit was equally effec-tive. These pH changes were quite significant. A living organism cannot survive the dramatic alterations of pH that these experiments induced. In two other experiments, they also altered, by programming intention devices, the *in vitro* function of the enzyme alkaline phosphatase and the ratio of ATP/ADP in fruit fly larvae, robustly affecting their rate of development into adults.

Tiller's conclusions from these experiments were far-reaching. He de-clared that the human aspects of thought, emotion, spirit, intention, and consciousness exist in the information wave aspect of his mathematical model. These human qualities in the information wave space can, under some circumstances, couple with the coarse particulate aspect of everyday reality and interact with it. Inner self-management, through meditation or other practices of the mind, spirit, and emotions, conditions the coupling between the two reciprocal spaces, thereby facilitating the availability of the information wave space to the master of such a practice.

Further, Tiller concluded that these information waves must exceed the speed of light, being the reciprocal of the particulate reality. Together the coarse particulate reality and the information wave reality add up, Tiller calculated, to the square of the speed of light, the last term in Einstein's famous equation, $E = mc^2$. Conservation of energy must take into account both the coarse particulate and the fine information wave aspects of this model. In other words, the activity of thought and physical reality must be taken together in the calculations using these new equa-tions. Thus, the particulate reality moves slower than the speed of light, and the information wave reality moves faster than the speed of light.

Tiller also asserted that the energy available in the information wave aspect is enormous; the energy available in the particulate space is a mere whisper by comparison. The space that exists within the atom and between atoms holds this enormous energy. The space between the nucleus and the orbiting electrons constitutes the vast majority of the atom. The greater density of the matter in the coarse particulate reality holds the ordinary amounts of energy with which we are familiar. He believed humanity will be able to tap these "vacuum energies" to our great benefit within the next decades. (See Section V.A: "Amrit Sorli" for more on vacuum energies.)

Leaving the programmed intention devices in a room for a few weeks to months, Tiller noticed an effect on the space itself. An oscillation developed in the room. He could measure oscillations of temperature, pH, and other factors whose fundamental frequencies nested in time and space. Even if he attempted to circulate the air with powerful fans blowing across the measuring devices to equilibrate the temperature, something more fundamental occurred to maintain oscillations of temperature and other factors. He theorized that the reciprocal space of the information wave pattern reality was being affected and the coupling between that space and the particulate space reality was facilitated by the length of time that the intention device was in the space. He was able to measure these effects for as much as one year after the intention device was removed. Perhaps Tiller had discovered the basic influence that drives oscillations that we find everywhere in nature, including the human body.

Tiller declared that this model of reality says that humans matter. With this perspective of reality, we could infer that humans are uniquely equipped to participate in creation. The coupling that occurs between the two realities offers the opportunity for human intention to affect the course of human events and the structure of physical reality. He asserted that healing occurs because of just such behavior. The healer and the one receiving the healing both access the other side (Divine, for Still) to return to a state of the "normal anatomy" (Still) or the form of the "morphic field" (Sheldrake).

Tiller's model is consistent with David Bohm's model of the implicate order (Tiller's information wave reality) and explicate order (Tiller's coarse particulate reality), although Bohm did not describe the human qualities of mind, emotions, and spirit with a concise mathematical model. Bohm indicated that these aspects could be accounted for by holomovement, the holographic creation of the explicate order from the implicate order.

What Tiller gave humanity is not only further evidence that there is a reality of Mind, as Still asserted, but also a means by which we can actually evaluate its effects quantitatively. Tiller mathematically proved Bohm's contentions, quantified the Taoists' empiric effectiveness, and explained in mathematical terms Benoit Mandelbrot and Rupert Sheldrake's theories. Tiller also added meat to the bones of osteopathic medicine's philosophy. Mind and Matter reciprocate to create the living form, to paraphrase Still.

Tiller's experiments demonstrated that Still's conception of Mind, Matter, and Motion was correct. Influenced by intention, alterations of pH and pK values affected developmental processes. In other words, Mind affected Motion in Matter. In Tiller's model, the information wave space is equivalent to Mind in Still's model, the coarse particulate space is equivalent to Matter, and the resultant of their "coupling" (Tiller's term) or the "connection between the physical and the spiritual" (Still's term) is biogen or life (Still). Intention influenced the developmental processes in Tiller's experiments and demonstrated the effects of Mind in form and motion, the two primary pieces of evidence of life in material substance.

The Wilkinson Microwave Anisotropy Probe (WMAP) is traveling in space about one million miles from Earth, sending back information about the formation and contents of the universe. "According to the probe, 4 percent of the universe is made up of ordinary matter . . . Twenty-three percent of the universe is made up of dark matter . . . The remainder of the universe, 73 percent, is what scientists call 'dark energy'."[36] This means that 96 percent of the universe is unknown. Is this unknown quantity what William Tiller and David Bohm theorized respectively, as "reciprocal space" and "implicate order"? Is dark matter and dark energy evidence of consciousness, that which underlies all of our ordinary reality? These are questions that some day we may have answers for.

III. SUMMARY OF MIND, MATTER, AND MOTION

The mind "thinks" with the body itself. — DAVID HAWKINS

To describe reality, all the philosophies and individuals mentioned so far used the following three elements: energy, matter, and life form. We can categorize the words used by each author or paradigm into these three categories, which we compare in Table 1 and review in the following list.

TABLE 1. **Comparison of Paradigms**			
Philosophy	**Energy**	**Matter**	**Life Form**
Still	Mind (Celestial)	Matter (Terrestrial)	Motion (life, spirit) Protoplasm (biogen)
Swedenborg	Soul (influx of spirit)	Body (invested in spirit)	Natural man
Chinese (Taoists)	Heaven	Earth	Evolution (life)
Native Americans	No-form	Form	Spirit
Sheldrake	Morphogenetic field	Material substance	Living form
Bohm	Implicate order	Explicate order	Form and motion
Tiller	Reciprocal space, information wave	Ordinary space, particulate matter	Oscillation in space

- Still indicated that biogen (form in motion) results from the union of the Celestial Father and the Terrestrial Mother.

- Swedenborg observed that the radiation from the Spiritual Sun, that is, the Love and Wisdom of God, harmonizes with its "cloak" of matter.

- The Taoists recognize *Qi* as the universal activating principle in their cosmology.

- Some Native Americans believe they are represented in No-form and are creating form from the earth.

- Sheldrake proposed morphogenetic fields to explain the derivation of form from a realm of energy that precedes material form.

- Bohm conceived in his model that consciousness is everywhere present, creating from the implicate order the explicate order with its form and motion.

- Tiller mathematically described two realities: the coarse particulate space and the information wave space.

The similarities of these cosmologies validate each other. They all point to the means by which life enters and manifests in physical reality. They imply that the life force is a substance that chooses its function and form in the material realm. These cosmologies all indicate there are two realities, one hidden and one material.

IV. STILL'S CLAIRVOYANCE AND SPIRITUALISM

By the law of knowledge and intuition all persons do succeed.

— A.T. STILL

"There are scores of well attested instances in which Dr. Still has shown his power of clairvoyance,—perhaps it would be better to say telepathy . . . In the case of Dr. Still, he seems to have inherited this power, if such a thing is possible, from both sides of his family" (Booth, 19).

Arthur G. Hildreth, DO, who grew up knowing Still as he began his work in Kirksville, wrote the following account of Still's clairvoyance: "After sitting down and waiting a few minutes, Dr. Still came in, and mother said to him, 'Doctor, I have a good friend who is a near neighbor of mine who is sick and I want to see if you can tell me what ails her.' Until my dying day I shall never forget the scene nor the impression made upon me, boy though I was. The morning was a bright, beautiful, sunshiny one, the weather was warm, and the west door of his office was open. He was standing just a few feet in front of where we were sitting. After mother's question, he turned and gazed out the door, seeming to be lost in thought for a few minutes. Then turning to us, he said: 'Why your friend has goiter and if you will have her come up here I will remove it.' Mother said: 'Yes but doctor, they are very poor people; how can they pay you?' He replied: "Her husband can haul me a load of wood, can't he?' Mother told him they would only be too glad to do so. The lady came to him and the goiter was entirely removed" (in Booth, 29).

From Harry L. Chiles, DO, comes this account: "I was in close contact with the Old Doctor quite frequently, as I worked in the office of *The Journal of Osteopathy* during my last year in college, and he took quite an interest in that publication. Dr. Still talked quite freely at times of his theories and of what he expected the osteopathic profession to do. No one of us since has ever thought as deeply as Dr. Still thought.

No one of us has had the imagination and followed through with work to prove or disprove theories as Dr. Still. It was the use of his intellect coupled with a will to work that made him great, for Dr. Still's life, above all things, was practical. He had the power of relaxation such as I have never known. The sensitiveness of his soul heard the guns and saw the ships afire at Manila Bay and at Santiago, Cuba, and he told that great battles were going on a day or two before the wires brought news to us. Then there may have been a doubt of his power, but radio now does it for us obtuse ones, evidently he did not need it. He believed that the mind might be trained to see beneath the surface, as the x-ray does, and may be his mind did this for him in some of his rapid diagnoses. He said to me, 'The x-ray by tremendously increasing the vibrations brings to light what is beneath the surface. Why can we not train our minds to do it?' In the light of present-day science, why should it be impossible? Dr. Still's life had taught him to depend on himself and not on outside aids" (in Hildreth, 444).

Still earnestly explained his obsession with the life force and how it related to Spiritualism:

(5) Let me say right here I feel as a hungry child seeking the milk of its mother's breast. I am hungry mentally, absolutely hungry beyond description to obtain a more thorough acquaintance with the substance or principle known as human life. This hunger has been with me many years. I have nothing so precious that I would not give to have it satisfied. I want an undebatable knowledge, a better acquaintance with life and whether it be a substance or a principle that contains the many attributes of mind, such as wisdom, memory, the power of reason, and an unlimited number of other attributes. *This short statement is to honestly acquaint you with my object in devoting all of my time, far beyond a quarter of a century, to the study of man, his form, and all his wisely adjusted parts, both mental and physical.* I have explored for a better knowledge upon this important subject. My daily prayer has

been 'Give me that knowledge that will light up the human body in whom we find a union of life with matter and the combined attributes of this union.' I have listened to the theologian. He theorizes and stops. I have listened to the materialist. He philosophizes and fails. I have beheld the phenomena given through the *spiritualist* medium. His exhibits have been *solace* and *comfort to my soul,* believing that he gives much, if not conclusive proof, that the constructor who did build man's body still exists in a form of higher and finer substances, after leaving the old body, than before. (Still, in Booth, 18–19; italics added)

Still's reference to Spiritualism opens the way to understand his conception of reality. As E. Crowell comments regarding Still's involvement with the practice of Spiritualism, "The spiritualist philosophy favored beliefs in the fatherhood of God and the brotherhood of man, immortality of the soul, spiritual intercourse, the ministry of the angels, eternal progression, and happiness for all; it rejected the traditional Christian beliefs of the Trinity, the divine inspiration of the Bible, the atonement, baptism, Sabbath observance, resurrection of the dead, and—as if this were not enough—the concepts of heaven and hell" (in Trowbridge, 108). Still may have attended séances, as he refered to the phenomena given through the spiritualist medium. These provided comfort to Still, as indicated by his own words. Adherents to Swedenborg's philosophy were active in Kansas as early as 1858. Still lived in Kansas from 1853 to 1875. Spiritualism grew out of the search for the soul, Swedenborgianism being an important stimulant to this trend (Trowbridge, 106–111, 196).

Still's search for the soul is evident in his fervent desire (expressed in the previous quotation) and in his philosophy of Osteopathy. Clearly, he believed that the soul continues to exist, whether invested with a physical form or not. Still was convinced that unseen patterns of information (consciousness) exist in life and death. For him, it was consciousness, or what Still called Mind, that governed the life form and allowed for communication beyond life. Still indicated that Mind operated throughout creation.

To repeat a previous quotation:

(6) Life surely is a very finely prepared substance, which is the all-moving force of Nature, or that force that moves all nature from worlds to atoms. (Still 1892, 256)

From this quotation, the comparison of Still's construction of reality with the Taoists and Bohm is clear.

A. Modern Views on Clairvoyance

1. Karl Pribram and Clairvoyance

Karl Pribram, a neuroscientist from Stanford University, theorized that holography determines the brain's function. In describing Pribram's work, J. Shimotsu wrote: "He combines brain research with theoretical physics, covers the areas of normal and paranormal perception, and takes things out of the supernatural and explains them as a part of nature . . . Dr. Pribram also suggested that if we saw reality without our mathematical computations performed by the brain, we would know a world in the frequency domain, without time or space, just events."[37] This is what Joseph Rael described from a Native American perspective. Shimotsu went on to say, "Because our brains are a part of the big hologram, they have access, under certain conditions, to all the information in the principles of control. If there is no time and space, there is no here or there; psychic occurrences and the supernatural can occur in nature" (126–127). In short, Pribram explained how clairvoyance is consistent with the laws of physics.

2. William Tiller and Clairvoyance

William Tiller described a reality of information wave space that he asserted contains generic thoughts belonging to no one. Coupling with this, information wave space from our ordinary reality of the coarse particulate space is facilitated by practices that strengthen inner management, such as meditation. If the coupling to this source of information is enhanced by such practices as meditation, we should become more intuitive. Knowledge of future events or events that are occurring in the present at a distance is available to anyone who accesses the information wave space. That is where time and space have no meaning. That is where clairvoyance happens; it's the realm of spirit. This is the realm of Still's Mind.

3. David Bohm and Clairvoyance

David Bohm took his theoretic model of implicate and explicate orders to the next level by saying that insight is the means by which one perceives the unmanifest. He said, however, that thought gets in the way. If we attempt to use *active* pursuit of the thought process to achieve knowledge about the unmanifest, we get blocked or confused because a drop of water cannot perceive the entire ocean, just as the thought cannot perceive the greater thought of the unmanifest. But the *passive* reception of information about the unmanifest routinely occurs through reflection, contemplation, and meditation. "The suggestion is that insight is an intelligence beyond any of the energies that could be defined in thought."[38]

4. Summary of Clairvoyance

Intelligence of insight transforms matter and clarifies thought, according to Bohm. Rael's vibrational perception is a passive way of existence; it is a way of being. The active thought process, on the other hand, is a way of doing or of having. Therefore, active thought becomes, as Rael put it, definition, or placement. Science, as it is commonly pursued, is doing; meditation is being. The difference between the two suddenly becomes abundantly evident when we consider the possible outcomes, as Joseph Rael asserted. Doing, rather than being, creates attachments and suffering, much as Buddhism teaches. Awareness of the vibration of everything is an act of being and not naming. Being human is defined by being, not just doing.

Coupled with intense study, Still used contemplation to arrive at his understanding of humans and the world. Still used his talent of clairvoyance to access the implicate order and gain his profound insight. His intimate relation with the quiet of nature at the frontier facilitated this process. Still's *Autobiography* contains many images of his visions through which he showed how he came to his understandings. It is as if he wanted us to have a deeper understanding of his process and to know that he had obtained his knowledge from the "other side." Sometimes readers of Still's *Autobiography* have interpreted these visions as colorful allegories, dismissing their importance. I contend that these visions represent the process of Dr. Still's mind and intuition at work and that he dared to reveal them because he knew this very truth: They would show us where he gained his knowledge from. The visions not only demonstrate to us how Still arrived at his profound understanding, they also honor intuition, dreaming, contemplation, and prayer in the production of insight. Insight is the originator of science. Einstein confirmed this for us when he said that dreams provided him with insights that preceded his mathematical proofs. Einstein said, "The fairest thing we can experience is the mysterious. It is the fundamental emotion which stands at the cradle of true science."[39]

As a Spiritualist, the "other side" seemed familiar to Still. For most of his contemporaries and for most of us today, it is less familiar. It is no wonder that many people, then and now, consider(ed) him a "crank" and that many offered prayers that he might recover his senses. "Bancroft, America's greatest historian says it is sometimes difficult to distinguish between fanaticism and the keenest sagacity. The crank of one age may be the sage of the next; therefore, it is not such a bad thing after all to be called a crank" (anonymous, "contributed by a friend," in Still 1908, 391).

Bohm explained, in terms of modern physics, this process of insight, information passively unfolding to awareness from the implicate order through contemplation. Quantum physics and related subjects, as described by Pribram and Bohm, are the very concepts that medicine is integrating today; this integration constitutes the major force behind the revolution in medicine. To characterize this revolution in terms of Still's philosophy, we can say that medicine is integrating spirit. Drew Still, ahead of his time, had already demonstrated how this works; his visions were evidence of how he accessed the implicate order for insight, for intelligent information about the nature of reality. Still drew from the ultimate source of intelligence to which Bohm and Pribram referred, and he showed us in his writings how to do it. Indeed, Drew Still was inspired.

V. SPIRIT INVESTS MATERIAL

Consciousness is the vital energy that both gives life to the body and survives beyond it in a different realm of existence. — DAVID HAWKINS

A. Amrit Sorli—Weight of Consciousness

Amrit Sorli, a researcher in physiology, has shown that the weight of a plant or an animal diminishes immediately at death when the living organism is contained so that it cannot exchange any material substance with its environment. He theorized that this change in weight corresponds to "vacuum energies" or "subtle energies" with which the organism is in active relation and that the organism finds essential to function. At death, this relationship is terminated and the energies are liberated, decreasing the weight of the body.[40] These findings support Bohm's, Tiller's, and Still's contentions that the life force (spirit) or consciousness is a "substance" containing mass.

B. Masaru Emoto—Message from Water

Masaru Emoto,[41–42] a Japanese researcher showed that water is a receptacle that receives spirit. He photographed small droplets of frozen water that had been exposed to different energetic influences while in the liquid state. The stunning results imply that thought, intention, and other vibrations such as music affect the crystallization of the water molecules to produce snowflake patterns or other disorganized photographic images according to the degree to which the vibration is harmonious with life.

In one set of experiments, he photographed samples of polluted water, which appeared as ugly and disorganized as we might expect fouled water to appear; in contrast, pure water from streams or springs appeared as beautiful crystalline structures resembling snowflakes. In another experiment, he photographed distilled water, which appeared to be without structural organization. However, after he placed various labels on vials of distilled water and left them overnight, the photographs taken the next day revealed the intention of the written words on the label: "Adolph Hitler" looked frighteningly ugly; "I hate you, I want to kill you" appeared similarly; "Thank you" appeared as a beautiful crystalline conformation as did "Mother Theresa." A third and most impressive experiment revealed that prayer offered over a vial of polluted water changed its photographic pattern from ugly and disorganized to that of a beautiful crystalline snowflake.

Such evidence helps explain the placebo effect, the expression in one's physiology of one's attitude, and the benefits of prayer. These experiments demonstrate for us in clear visual terms how "mind over matter" works. These observations of water have far-reaching implications that deserve serious and rigorous study.

This work directly applies to Still's philosophy because it demonstrates that form develops from unseen influences, including thought, intent, and prayer. Further, it is clear that water is a receptacle for these influences. Further still, it can be seen that these influences create symmetry and beauty when they are consistent with life, health, and love; the reverse is also true, that the influences create asymmetry and ugliness when they are not consistent with life, health, and love. These influences are similar in effect to the life essence that Still (and the others we have mentioned) postulated to create form and Motion in Matter from an influence of Mind.

C. Theodor Schwenk—Living Water

In his marvelous book, *Sensitive Chaos* (1996),[43] Theodor Schwenk developed his ideas about the nature of water and its formative impulse with illustrations to prove how its vitality produces patterns of life. Injecting into still water another stream of water from a pipe or needle, Schwenk created flows of intermingling water that resembled embryonic forms. These displays of nature's formative spirit offer compelling evidence that water carries out the impulse to create a material "cloak" for an unseen life essence.

Schwenk went on to say that, while solid *objects* impose themselves on space and exclude other structures from the same space, *movement* can be multiple and diverse within one space. This is demonstrated when waves in a body of water that are coming from different directions meet at one place. Of course, we see multiple and diverse wave patterns in the human body manifested as blood, lymph, cerebrospinal fluid, and extracellular and intracellular fluid dynamics. Multiple movements,

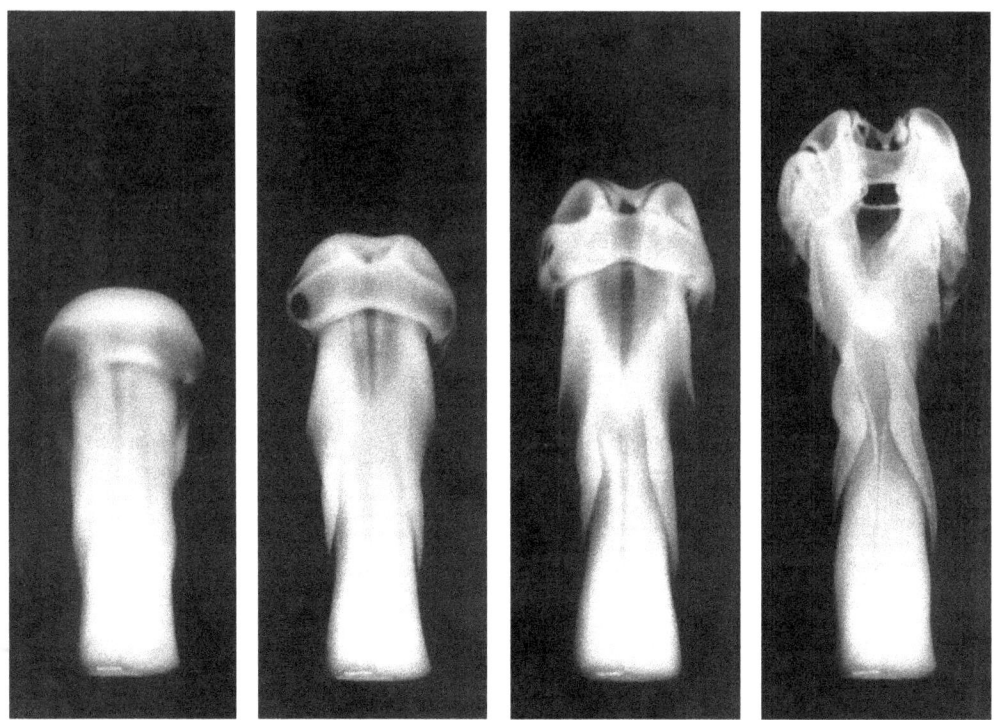

2.6 Natural conformations resembling embryos, generated from dyed water injected into still water. (Reproduced with permission from PLATES 49–54, in the gallery of plates in Schwenk T (1996). *Sensitive Chaos*. 2nd Ed. London: Rudolf Steiner Press.)

vibrations, rhythms, and fluctuations occur in the same space, interpenetrating each other. Therefore, movement is seen to be independent of space; although appearing in a space, it acts as a regulating principle of that space (Schwenk, 28–29).

Two obvious forms of waves occur in water: (1) passing waves on the surface of still water, in which the energy of the wave creates a crest and a trough as it passes but the molecules of the surface water are relatively stationary, describing an ellipse as the wave rises and falls; and (2) standing waves, for instance behind a rock in a stream, in which the wave is stationary but the molecules of water move through it. A third, less obvious type of wave is expressed in bodies of water as described by Schwenk: "Every water basin, whether ocean, lake or pond, has its

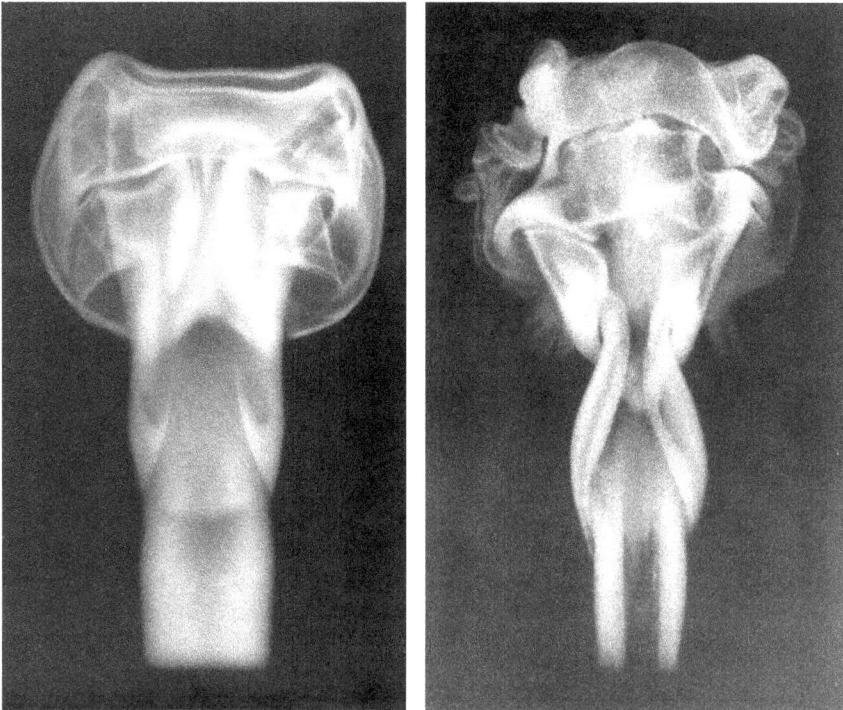

own natural period of vibration . . . It is like a 'note' to which the lake is 'tuned'" (30). Like pushing a child on a swing, the effects of the pull of the moon as it circles around the Earth or of a change in atmospheric pressure might create a harmonic with this note and facilitate its amplitude. This effect is called the "tide."

Schwenk goes on to say: "The creation of form in living substance is only thinkable if manifold movements can flow into, over, and through one another at one and the same place in space. The fluid element is thus a most suitable medium for the form-creating process, which would be impossible in the three-dimensional world of solids, where there is only exclusiveness and no interpenetration . . . [Movements] appear in the spatial world as though from higher realms and in so doing create law and order . . . In the hen's egg the inner formative processes in the embryo are accompanied by rhythmical wave movements. These run in a gentle wave of contractions over the amnion of the egg from one end to the other and back" (Schwenk, 34).

Inner surfaces are formed in a body of water if parts of the volume flow at different rates, as in a pipe or stream, or if there are other irregularities of temperature or of content, such as electrolytes. If rates of flow are greatly disparate, turbulence results. The inner surfaces behave in a sentient manner creating vortices and tend to roll one layer in on the other. "In short, wherever the finest differentiations are present the water acts as a delicate 'sense organ' which as it were perceives the differentiations and then in a rhythmical process causes them to even out and to merge" (Schwenk, 39).

As soon as different media flow together, for instance warm and cold water, the one is taken into the other so that a hollow space is formed and, like a vessel, is filled with a fluid of a different quality. This new fluid is created out of the action of the two mingling liquids. The creation of the hollow form is an archetypal process that can be found everywhere in nature. The gastrulation process in embryogenesis is an outstanding example of such an act of creation in which a unique quality is captured in the enfolding fluid and can take on a life of its own. "Boundary surfaces, with their rhythmical processes, are birthplaces of living things. It is as though the creative, formative impulse *needed* the boundary surfaces in order to be able to act in the material world. Boundary surfaces are everywhere the places where living, formative processes can find a hold; be it in cell membranes, surfaces of contact *between* cells, where the life forces are mysteriously present" (Schwenk, 41–42).

As we will see, the human "body of water" also has an inherent rhythm, like the standing wave in the stream. The container of this body of water, the connective tissues, holds an inherent resonance peculiar to this particular type of form and this particular specimen. We can generalize and state that all form is moment by moment being created by movement, with a constant stream of substance flowing through it. Organic form, in spite of the continuous exchange of material, remains intact. The fact that forms remain intact despite continuous exchange with their environment is evidence that an energy pattern holds the form. The human form, like a standing wave in a stream, holds its form because of a pattern of energy that retains its shape despite a constant exchange of material with its environment. Clearly, form comes from vibration, from an unseen pattern. Just as the rock in the stream creates a standing wave, so too there is a force that creates the standing wave of human form. The pattern for the human form derives from an archetypal map or design that exists in a hidden realm. This design couples with flowing substance in the visible realm. Because the pattern is vibration and the flow of substance is movement, oscillation is detectable everywhere and at every level we might investigate. Thus, a tide is evident in a watery matrix, even a human matrix.

D. Erich Blechschmidt—Embryology

Erich Blechschmidt[44] declared, after decades of careful embryological observation that the human form derives from influences that come from outside as much as those that come from within the developing embryo. He stated that genetic activity can be reactive as well as proactive and that mechanical forces outside of or on the surface of the developing embryo can direct the course of the development of the embryo with as much certainty as genes or metabolism. In fact, early metabolic activity of the embryo consists of the interaction of the surface of the embryo and the maternal uterine lining. With implantation, the degeneration of the endometrium occurs due to the embryo's invasion. This material from the degeneration of maternal tissue feeds the embryo. This important first interaction with its environment assures the embryo's survival.

Intrinsic metabolic and genetic directives not only have impacts on but also are impacted by conformational aspects of development. For example, in some cases, flows of metabolic fluids determine the relative sizes of developing structures. Further, genetics does not drive development until individual characteristics (hair and eye color, size of nose, etc.) begin to be incorporated into the basic superstructure of the common embryological morphology.

What is even more interesting is that the embryo acquires space from the surrounding fluid medium in order to grow rather than growing solely by the process of cellular multiplication and expansion from within. At the end of a limb bud, for example, the embryo first establishes influence over the space into which it will grow within the fluid medium. Then it sends its multiplying cells into the appropriated space. The form is first created in fluid; the material body follows. Thus, a pattern of energy advances before the expanding cellular encroachment into the extra-embryonic fluid environment as the limb bud forms. This is an important sequence determining form: first energy, then fluid, and then cellular structure. This sequence describes the manner by which the form is maintained, as well. Energy exists as a pattern from which water receives the information and passes it on to the connective tissues that establish the form in three-dimensional physical reality. The vibration of these three aspects of the system—energy, water, and solid substance—is essential for the maintenance of the form.

This picture developed by Blechschmidt is one in which the embryo reacts to and derives its form within the context of its environment. In this manner, Blechschmidt added to our understanding of the holographic nature of the developing embryo. In this view, the human form develops from its surroundings. It is a part of All-That-Is. Therefore, we have further evidence of the manner by which Mind and Matter interact to create form. In embryology, we see this action of Mind with Matter most immanently. The developing embryo is the quintessential example of the creation of form from undifferentiated matter.

1. Biogen in Embryology

To translate the term "biogen" into a term that is more commonly used today, we might choose the word "protoplasm." In fact, Hulett and Booth, two writers about Still's philosophy who worked with him, penned the term "protoplasm" in reference to biogen. Furthermore, Still also used the word "protoplasm" in his later writing. As we know, undifferentiated protoplasm is tissue whose form and function are yet to be determined. It is pluripotent, formless, and it is prepared for whatever assignment it receives. This protoplasm is Matter in Motion (living tissue) that has not yet received its instructions from Mind. It is the raw essence of life that has been invested in its most elementary material preparation. It is the tissue from which differentiation emerges to fulfill the demands placed on it by function. The function is determined by Mind, and the form is determined by the function. Form, once established, can also determine function. Therefore, both form and function result from Mind's interaction with Matter. This is precisely how Still described the formation of biogen, that is, Mind and Matter reciprocating to create form in Motion. Form in Motion is biogen, the basic building block of living tissue.

2. Health and Biogen

Biogen contains health. "Health" used in this particular context denotes more than a description of a condition. It is a nominative expression of force and power moving through the system. Disturbed or distorted tissue contains less health, and health comes into the tissue when its conformation is normalized to permit it. If the structure of the tissue represents the original, then the permitted function also represents the original. James Jealous, DO,[45] described healing as a return to the original. The return to the original is a resumption of the morphic field and the movement of *Qi*, which defines the form and function of health. If we can find the health, as Still exhorted us to do, rather than naming the disease, then healing occurs as a function of the protoplasm. The biogen has within it the impetus to heal. Striking clinical results, often beyond ordinary expectations, follow such a simple but profound approach.

VI. SYNTHESIS AND LOOKING AHEAD

Do not seek to follow in the footsteps of the wise; seek what they sought.
— AUTHOR UNKNOWN

From the original concepts that Dr. Still enunciated, to the most ancient and aboriginal ideas, to the most modern thoughts of new physics, we have a concurrence of ideas. How do these congruent systems of thought from disparate sources advance our understanding of Still's philosophy? We can synthesize these views as follows.

1. Creation consists of two dynamics: the life force and material substance.
2. These two reciprocate to produce a living form in motion.
3. The unseen pattern of the life force, directed by consciousness, permeates the substance of the earthly material to enliven it with thought, emotion, metabolism, and behavior.
4. The visible earth-based material returns to a state of lesser activity unless the vitalizing principle of the soul continues to course through it.
5. Fluids are the medium for the transmission of the life force within material substance—thus the importance of the circulation of blood in Osteopathy.

We readily differentiate between greater and lesser vitalizing activity in the human when we observe a sleeping individual and compare it to a corpse. We also observe the beginnings of this difference when we palpate normal tissue and compare it to injured tissue. The injured tissue is less vital, less imbued with health, less compatible with life; and, if left unchanged, it will progress to develop conditions of disease and to distribute these adverse effects to farther reaches through its connections through nerves, vessels, and connective tissues. Pain and disability mark this progression toward disease of the injured area. Vitality, called health, cannot penetrate the region as it did in its original conformation. If the original shape of the area is reestablished, health returns and recovery is possible.

Bone and the other connective tissues transduce the impulse generated by morphic fields to determine the shape of the body. The connective tissues are the container for the fluids that carry the life force. If the fluids that carry health penetrate the tissues freely, the organism is healthy. If there is energetic or conformational distortion changing its original shape, then the health is less available and the condition of the organism declines. So, the objective of osteopathic treatment is to assist the organism from the outside in order to facilitate the connective tissues to restore themselves from the inside to their original conformation and to allow optimal health. Because the structural element of the body often requires assistance from outside to regain its original conformation, osteopathic manipulative medicine exists.

The preexisting functional element created the original conformation of the parts and the whole organism in the embryo. The exuberant forces of embryogenesis occur on a tiny scale in a mostly fluid medium, facilitating the generation of the original form. However, once the form is firmly established in connective tissue matrices, it will not easily remodel when deformed. This is especially true if the sole influence for remodeling is the energy of the function for which the structure was created. If the matrix is distorted, this functional activity, which is no longer equipped to generate form, also has to contend with a much larger mass of a much tougher tissue than the forces of embryogenesis did. In fact, the function itself, within this distorted form, has a reduced ability to deal with remodeling because the conformation change has reduced its potency. Thus, restoring full function depends on restoring the container of the function to its original shape. Then, the fluids can carry the life force and nutrition unimpeded throughout the organism.

The fluids of the body circulate and fluctuate. Circulation depends on vascular and neural integrity. Fluctuation or oscillation depends on the expression of the original conformation of the connective tissue. Vascular and neural functions also require that there be free movement of their respective activities without interference from distorted connective tissue. Oscillation is inherent in fluid containers, especially between compartments with electrochemical concentration gradients.

Not only does the life force create the form and then vivify it, it is directed by consciousness as a carrier of thought and intention. The purpose of being has as much to do with health as does the condition of the physical structure. In fact, the material from which the structure derives responds to thought and intention as much as it does to nutrition and the life force. The connective tissues are both electrical and mechanical, that is, piezoelectric. The shape of the connective tissue transduces a pattern of preexisting energy that determines its shape in the embryo, but the adult shape also depends on this influence to maintain its health. The connective tissues transduce these and other forces that regularly impact it, such as trauma, thoughts, and emotions. Over time, the more subtle effects from thoughts express themselves in the mechanical structure of the organism. Disturbances of posture, mobility, and organ function result not only from injury, illness, and habits of drink and food but also from thought and intention.

Moreover, thought, prayer, and purpose affect others as well as each of us as individuals. As a society or individually, we experience influences with no outwardly apparent cause that affect our health. Special attention to these subtleties carries a responsibility that Native Americans live out in their paradigm. Mainstream medicine and the dominant American society blatantly disregard any notion that subtle energies could play a significant role in the production or maintenance of illness or in everyday physical, emotional, or mental responses of individuals and populations. "Mind over matter" is a verity that needs and deserves our attention and respect. The next step in medicine will honor this aspect and use it to the benefit of all humans. We will learn about it by studying the placebo effect. The next step in medicine will unify ancient and modern, mental and physical. Osteopathic medicine is uniquely prepared through its heritage to accept this challenge.

3

EXPLORATIONS INTO
THE LIFE FORCE

This chapter explores what we know about the life force or vital force in the human body, which is fundamental to Andrew Taylor Still's philosophy and to this book. First, we look at original osteopathic writings for references to the life force. Then, we move to perhaps the best-known proponent of the vital force in osteopathic medicine, William Garner Sutherland, DO, reviewing his life and research. Finally, our exploration takes us to others outside the profession who comment about that which provides vitality to living organisms and the mechanisms of that vital force in the physical.

I. REFERENCE TO THE LIFE FORCE IN OSTEOPATHIC TEXTS

To research this subject, we first revisit how the concept of the life force was treated within the early osteopathic profession once Dr. Still had planted the seed. Most osteopathic writers, such as C. Hazzard (1900),[1] M. A. Lane (1918),[2] and C. P. McConnell and C. C. Teall (1920),[3] neglected to mention the vital force in their texts in reference to the osteopathic philosophy. Carl McConnell, DO, and Charles Hazzard, DO, who sequentially held the post of Professor of Osteopathic Practice at the American School of Osteopathy (ASO), did not develop the concept of the life force in their books. In fact, Still commented that McConnell's textbook, *The Practice of Osteopathy* (1899), referenced many "old medical authors," making it useless for osteopaths. This fact may have added further inspiration for Still to write his own books.[4] What's more, Hazzard's books were his collected lectures at the ASO from 1898 to 1900, and they were devoid of spiritual references. We might conclude from this fact that A. T. Still's was the lone voice at the ASO that spoke about the life force in relation to Osteopathy.

However, in an article that McConnell authored in the *Journal of the American Osteopathic Association* (JAOA) (1913),[5] he alluded to spirit, mentioning that the evolutionist Herbert Spencer's definition of life was illuminating: "the continuous adjustment of internal relations to external relations." McConnell went on, "The best we can do is to keep the mechanism intact anatomically, physiologically, and environmentally so that the life-giving protecting forces may continue to act . . . We call it scientific because it is true, and it is true because it succeeds" (McConnell, 504). But, although this quotation alludes to a life force relative to the body's structure and function, demonstrating that it appears as a practical truth, McConnell does not go so far as to make a strong statement advocating, as Still did, that the life force is fundamental in the osteopathic philosophy.

Further, the weakening position of the subject of the life force in the osteopathic philosophy is evident in the early faculty at the ASO. Still recruited from other educational institutions some of the important figures on the faculty in the early years of the ASO. "In 1897, Dr. Still added the following individuals to his staff: D. M. Desmond, PhD, a graduate of both Harvard University and the Baltimore Medical College (physiology); C. W. Proctor, DO, a graduate of Allegheny College in Pennsylvania with postgraduate work at the University of Berlin, Germany (chemistry); Charles Hazzard, DO, a graduate of Northwestern University and also the ASO (histology and later, principles of osteopathy); A. H. Sippey, MD, PhD (urinalysis)"[6] and others. These individuals began to emphasize the success of the college and their careers, even to the point of sacrificing the osteopathic philosophy and favoring the introduction of *materia medica* (use of drugs) into the curriculum.

Things came to a head in 1899 when Still appointed A. G. Hildreth, DO, the dean. Because they claimed Hildreth was "ultra-osteopathic," several of the faculty resigned, including William Smith, who had helped found the ASO in 1892. Hildreth did not have an advanced degree beyond high school, unlike many of the faculty under his control. His appointment to the position of dean pitted the highly educated, conventionally trained faculty from the East against the *de novo* approach to healing that Still had developed on the frontier as a purely osteopathic perspective. Later, Still was quoted as saying, "We have no further use for the East," referring to his desire to have a purely American institution "uncluttered with terminology derived from foreign languages" (in Trowbridge, 155).

It is interesting to note that Hildreth was in the first class at the ASO, the class that nearly ended Still's attempts to train others in his method. Still felt he had failed to impart to them the necessary information and techniques to become adequate "osteopathists." He had wondered if his method could be taught, if others could learn to use the healing capacity in the body, but he recognized that some members of his family had been able to learn Osteopathy and to help him with the overflow of patients pouring into Kirksville. At the advice of a respected friend and clergyman, Still chose his next classes more carefully to assure their scholarly ability, and he lengthened the curriculum to two years. He also recruited skilled faculty to teach additional subjects of a more technical nature, the same faculty that now had begun to question whether Still's original hypothesis was acceptable in conventional medical circles.

It is also interesting to note that Hildreth was very loyal to Still. He later wrote, in *The Lengthening Shadow of Dr. A. T. Still* (1938),[7] how he had deeply admired Still from his childhood on. Still appointed Hildreth because he knew that he would continue the method of the "Old Doctor" in the midst of the many attempts to undercut it.

There was ample evidence of many attempts to change Osteopathy or to usurp the power that had coalesced around Still and his new

3.1 Officers, teachers, and operators, ASO, 1897. (Reproduced from the *Journal of Osteopathy*, 1897.)

school. Many new graduates chartered other osteopathic schools around the country, thirteen being established between 1896 and 1899, some of which became diploma mills and one of which sat across the street from the ASO. One institution, started by Elmer Barber in Kansas City (1895) even claimed to have originated Osteopathy. A magnetic healer, D. D. Palmer, came to Kirksville in 1893. He returned to his home a short distance north of Kirksville, in Davenport, Iowa, announcing his discovery of Chiropractic in 1895. He named his new profession after the Greek word for hand, *chiro*, and started a school in 1898. Three brothers, J. Martin, James, and David Littlejohn, wanted to expand the teachings of Osteopathy, even demanding that the ASO grant them an MD degree. When the conflict with Still reached its peak, they instituted legal action against Still and started their own osteopathic college in Chicago, The American School of Osteopathic Medicine and Surgery, in 1900. The American Association for the Advancement of Osteopathy (AAAO), which was renamed the American Osteopathic Association (AOA) in 1901, advocated a broadened osteopathic approach following the lead of the Littlejohns.

In addition, the new, highly trained faculty that Still had hired attempted to introduce *materia medica* into the curriculum. They perceived that the success of the new institution that employed them depended on standards with which they were familiar, those of medical institutions in the eastern United States and Europe. Thus, very early in the development of the profession, there was already strong evidence of the attempts by others to gain power and to move away from Still's original ideas.

Hildreth's loyalty as dean to continue the thread of Still's philosophy as Still became older (now 71 years) became essential. After all, Hildreth was succeeding as the first lobbyist of the profession. He convinced legislators, often by treating them, to vote for the acceptance of Osteopathy. He designed legislation for several states that were the first to legally accept Osteopathy (Trowbridge, 141–194).

During this time, A. T. Still continued to be quite active at the institution. He taught osteopathic philosophy and technique and regularly entered various classes unannounced to set a lecturer straight or to give his view of the osteopathic philosophy through storytelling, demonstration, or allegory. Despite his influence, the trend to exclude the life force as a part of the osteopathic philosophy continued in succeeding years. Writings by G. J. Conley (1935),[8] A. G. Hildreth (1938), and H. E. Litton (1944)[9] provide ample evidence for this. These authors preferred to describe osteopathic technique and to leave the philosophy largely unwritten.

However, at least two authors, G. D. Hulett (1903)[10] and E. R. Booth (1905)[11] discussed biogen, protoplasm, the life force, and/or the vital force in their books (see Chapters One and Two). Hulett succeeded Hazzard and McConnell as Professor of Osteopathic Practice at the ASO. Like many of the other members of the faculty who had advanced degrees, Hulett held BS and DO degrees and Booth held PhD and DO degrees. These authors distinguished themselves from the rest by writing about philosophy as well as technique.

After these writings of Booth and Hulett in the early years of the twentieth century, it was not until *The Cranial Bowl*[12] was published (1939) that an osteopathic physician fully acknowledged the vital force as a fundamental aspect of the osteopathic philosophy. William Garner Sutherland, DO, DSc (Hon) (1873–1954) independently described what he called the "Breath of Life," a term he abstracted from Genesis 2:7 in the Bible: "And the Lord God formed man of the dust of the ground, and breathed into his nostrils the *breath of life*; and man became a living soul" [italics added].

His own discovery of the Breath of Life, began with his brilliant observation of the potential for motion in the human skull. Subsequent to this observation, he spent the rest of his years and his osteopathic career investigating, discovering, and characterizing the manifestations of the Breath of Life (the life force). He first worked with bony specimens and

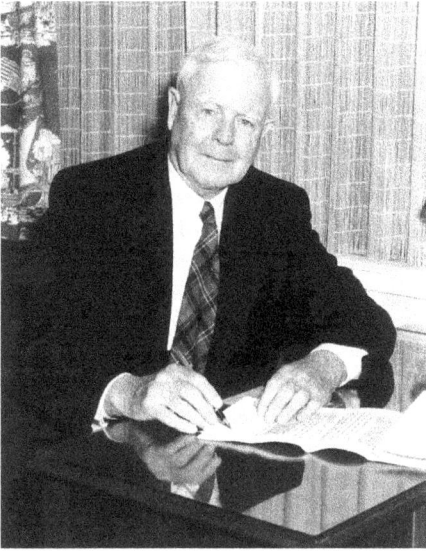

3.2   W. G. Sutherland, DO, signing the Articles of Incorporation of the Sutherland Cranial Teaching Foundation, 1953.

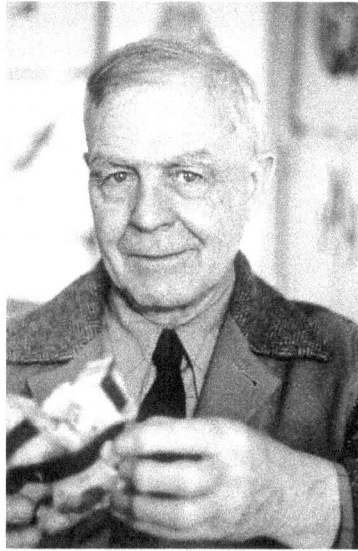

3.3   W. G. Sutherland, DO, holding a sphenoid bone.

his own living skull. Next, he applied these discoveries to his patients in treatment, realizing undeniable benefits. Eventually, he began teaching other osteopathic physicians how to treat using the Breath of Life, some forty years after his original insight.

He asserted that the Breath of Life engenders a subtle, palpable oscillation, which he called the "primary respiratory mechanism," a discovery that someday may be viewed for what it is, one of the most outstanding contributions in the history of physiology. This subtle motion is found in the tissues of the central nervous system (the brain and spinal cord); in the potent, nutritive, and protective fluid that it produces (the cerebrospinal fluid); in the container of the CNS (the dura mater and other meninges, skull, spine, and sacrum); and in all the other organs and tissues of the body.

II. THE STORY OF WILL SUTHERLAND

Will Sutherland was a student at the ASO in Kirksville, Missouri, at the turn of the century, when much was happening. Still had just published his *Autobiography* (1898), the new Infirmary had been completed (1895) and then expanded (1896), the American Association for the Advancement of Osteopathy had been formed (1897), and the *Journal of Osteopathy* (1894) was being published. Still was very interested in the development of all of these institutions. At age 70, he was actively involved in teaching when Will Sutherland entered the ASO in 1898, six years after the school's first charter had been approved.

When he was twenty-five, Will decided to leave the newspaper career that he had begun as a teenager in South Dakota and Minnesota to study Osteopathy. He chose Osteopathy after visiting the ASO with a friend, Herschel Conner, from Austin, Minnesota, who preceded Sutherland at the institution by one year. Sutherland's visit came after he had also been convinced that there was something to Osteopathy, having observed improvement in his brother's health from osteopathic treatment and after meeting A. T. Still's son, Charles, who had just opened a new practice in Red Wing, Minnesota.

A. A Guiding Thought

Will Sutherland enrolled at the ASO and was taught by Still, among others, but in a student body of over seven hundred, he did not develop a personal relationship with the "Old Doctor." In fact, Still admonished the graduates of that time to not claim themselves to be favorites of Dr. Still but to take their diplomas as sufficient evidence of their education and adequacy as a practitioner of Osteopathy.

Sutherland commented, however, that he had received personal instruction from Still. At times, Still placed his hands on Sutherland's hands to demonstrate a point of treatment. The Old Doctor's words surely captured and stimulated Sutherland's mind. Evidence of this permeates Sutherland's ideas and writing. Howard Lippincott, a student of William Sutherland wrote: "At the time that Dr. Sutherland received his osteopathic training at Kirksville, Dr. Andrew Taylor Still was carefully supervising all the instruction given at the college. The principles that were taught had to conform exactly to his concept. Dr. Sutherland made good use of every opportunity to learn and understand them and has adhered closely in his thinking and practice to Dr. Still's principles throughout his professional career. In consequence the technique which he has presented to us is a reflection of the clear vision of our founder."[13]

So, Sutherland served as a bridge for Still's philosophy from the time that Still's teaching declined at Kirksville in the first decade of the twentieth century to the time when Sutherland introduced the cranial concept to the osteopathic profession in the 1930s. Sutherland repeatedly expressed to his students that what he was teaching them was Still's philosophy. He often quoted Still and directed his students "to read between the lines" of Still's writings to find the meaning that he, Sutherland, was bringing forward. Sutherland denied that the cranial concept originated with him; in the same manner, Still had said that Osteopathy was a child of the Mind of God and that he, Still, was grateful to have merely discovered it.

Still's concepts of Osteopathy certainly were in Sutherland's mind when he was walking between classes, as he frequently did in the old North Hall, during his second and last year in 1899. On one occasion, as he passed by a glass case displaying Still's bony specimens, his attention was drawn to the bones of the skull. The particular skull on display held the bones in correct relationship, but separated from each other to reveal the sutures more clearly. He found the sphenosquamous suture especially compelling. Recalling this experience, he was quoted as saying: "As I stood looking and thinking in the channel of Dr. Still's philosophy, my attention was called to the beveled articular surfaces of the sphenoid bone. Suddenly there came a thought—I call it a guiding thought—'beveled, like the gills of a fish, indicating articular mobility for a respiratory mechanism.' "[14]

B. A Crazy Thought

Immediately, he thought, "How crazy can a fellow's thinking get? Mobility? In the bones of the skull? A dome such as that?" (Sutherland A, 13) As incongruous as the thought was, nevertheless it intrigued him. And the thought kept repeating itself in his head. After graduating in June 1900, he turned to his new practice and continued pushing the idea of skull mobility out of his mind. But eventually the tasks at hand slowed enough for him to ask, "But why that beveling, if not for a purpose? Couldn't that purpose be provision for movement?" (Sutherland A, 13)

He began to speculate about how he could go about proving to himself that what he had been taught was true: "That the bones of the skull do not move." Then, he dared to entertain the corollary question, how could he prove to himself, for his own peace of mind, that there was indeed mobility of the bones of the skull. But he scolded himself with the thought, "Why I'd be a ridiculous Don Quixote attempting to tilt an anatomical belief centuries old. If such an idea is as irrational as it seems to be, what might that indicate regarding me?" (Sutherland A, 15) After all, Will Sutherland was a quiet and retiring man, not bent on making waves.

C. Get Going

Finally, as the years passed and Sutherland became settled in his new practice, his curiosity could no longer be contained, and he said to himself, "Quit hedging and get going!" He determined that he must examine the sutures, which would require a disarticulated skull. He used what he had at hand—his ingenuity, curiosity, the intact skull he had brought from Kirksville that he called "Mike," and his penknife. So, he began to work to separate the bones with the knife, a daunting and nearly impossible task. Not only did he succeed in disarticulating the skull, he also was able to fashion the parts so that they could be rejoined, using special clips and bands to reassemble them.

D. Bony Motion

Like Andrew Still before him, Will Sutherland examined the bones. Because structure follows function, he reasoned, the underlying physiology had created their form. He realized that the bones could reveal to him secrets of their formation like rocks do to a geologist. Impressions from the effects of fluids, wind and water, tell a story about the rocks. So too, the vascular and cerebrospinal fluids, as well as the soft brain, itself, left impressions for Sutherland's inquisitive mind. Most important, he recognized that the sutures themselves were molded by fluid activity as revealed in the reciprocal beveling of each suture where two bones meet.

The beveling of the sutures told him of minute motions between the bones. He found evidence of gliding movements, rotations, rocking, and shuttle movements among others. From simply examining the conformation of the sutures, he began to piece together the motion patterns of single bones, then to relate how each bone moves with its neighbors, and eventually to visualize the motion of the whole skull. The patterns within each suture that he discovered were consistent from specimen to specimen. Detailed descriptions of each suture and its implied motions can be found in *Osteopathy in the Cranial Field* by Harold Magoun, DO.[15–16]

Gradually, Sutherland confirmed for himself that the standard texts were wrong about the closure of the sutures. They said that the sutures of the skull begin to ossify at about the age of forty years and that they continue to fuse until about the eightieth year. Sutherland countered with this comparison: "The trunk of the mighty oak possesses flexibility to a certain degree until it becomes a sapless log. The same may be said of the flexibility of the skull, as long as the sap remains." He went on to say, "We are too prone to accept the version of the authorized texts and reason from the cold cadaver" (Sutherland A, 21).

Once again, Sutherland was taking after his mentor, Still, by daring to step outside the accepted norms of thought. He dared to conclude that conventional thought held errors that undermined its applied effectiveness. He explained that medical authorities may not have all the answers and that original thinking was required for the advancement of the discipline. One physician from the establishment, Fritz Kahn, who authored the popular two-volume set, *Man in Structure and Function* (1943), agreed with Sutherland's concepts. Kahn wrote, "The bones of the skull do not grow together and unite, but instead they develop zig-zag sutures which dovetail together in an interlocking joint. These zig-zag sutures hold the bones firmly together while at the same time permitting a very slight degree of mobility."[17]

1. References against Cranial Mobility

The commonly held belief that there is fusion of the sutures that prevents any cranial bone mobility arose in the mid-1900s. However, the authorities that are quoted as proof of this actually came to the opposite conclusions. References to cranial bone immobility often cite papers by Todd and Lyon, published in 1924 and 1925,[18–21] and other anthropologists. Ashley-Montagu (1938),[22] Singer (1953),[23] and Hershkovitz (1997)[24] all declared that one cannot relate chronological age to suture closure.

In all of these anthropological studies, the authors were hoping to correlate suture closure with the chronological age of the individual skull as a means of routinely aging archeological specimens. They all concluded that no correlation exists between suture closure and the chronological age of the individual. In fact, these authorities found that no matter what the age of the specimen, most skulls demonstrated *no* suture closure at all. The closure of sutures, in many cases, was and is simply structural evidence of pathological trauma.

Nevertheless, the impression became set in the minds of the medical profession and the public that, in adulthood, the skull is fused into one piece. To eradicate this thought seems to be as hard as the skull they imagine—it is all very fixed. But such a rigid skull is incompatible with life and health. It must have been this realization that drove Sutherland to risk his reputation, as contrary to his retiring personality and tendency to avoid controversy as it was.

2. Evidence for Mobility

Recent research clearly shows mobility is the norm in human skulls. Hollis King's paper, in *The Cranial Letter* (1999)[25] provides us with a good review of the scientific and medical literature that supports cranial bone mobility. One of the earliest papers to recognize sutural mobility was authored by Pritchard (1956).[26] The closure of sutures in rats and humans seems to be under the influence of various unphysiological events, according to a series of papers (1959, 1960) by Moss.[27–30]

Frymann (1971)[31] used calipers on the cranium to demonstrate motion relative to cardiac and respiratory activity, as well as a previously unrecorded third motion, slightly slower than pulmonary respiration. Hubbard (1971)[32–33] determined that cranial sutures demonstrate more compliance than layered cranial bones do. And St. Pierre and associates (1976)[34] described movement across sutures via changes of capacitance in metal plates positioned on either side of a suture.

Retzlaff and colleagues,[35] in a series of experiments at Michigan State

University in the 1970s, showed that the histological construction of adult sutures specifically accommodates subtle motion. The only change with increasing age, detected in one study, was a decrease in the number of collagenous fibers in the sutures.[36] Within the sutures are elements of connective tissue, vessels, and nerves. There is no bone-to-bone fusion,[37] although Sharpey's fibers are found binding the bones together in the sutural ligaments.[38] Because remodeling of bone is a normal process, especially at the margins of the sutures, it could give the appearance to histologists that this activity represents sutural closure.[39] Retzlaff demonstrated that sutures are patent in macaques[40] and squirrel monkeys[41] and that motion exists in the skulls of squirrel monkeys.[42]

Kokich (1976)[43] demonstrated that suture closure is not completed in the human even by the age of ninety-five. Adams and colleagues (1992)[44] showed that the phenomenon of cranial bone mobility exists in cats. Moskalenko and colleagues (1996, 1998)[45–47] used bioimpedence technology to demonstrate skull motion in the living human. They reported oscillations of the skull bones at frequencies of 6–14 cycles per minute.

Heisey and Adams, in a landmark paper (1993),[48] proved that the Monro-Kellie doctrine is false. In their paper, they referred to the Monro-Kellie "hypothesis"—downgrading it from a "doctrine"—the standard by which neurosurgeons had been calculating intracranial pressures. These calculations had been based on the assumption that the skull is rigid and therefore contains a constant volume of blood. Heisey and Adams showed that the skull indeed demonstrates compliance, the ratio of volume changes to pressure changes. Further, they demonstrated that this compliance is based, in part, on the movement of the cranial bones at their sutures.

Moskalenko and associates (1998)[49] duplicated the findings of Heisey and Adams with bolus injections into the carotid arteries and measured concurrent changes in cross-sectional dimensions of the human skull in the frontal and sagittal planes. Using sequential x-rays and nuclear magnetic resonance (NMR) tomograms, they also detected variations in these dimensions without bolus injections. These variations occur naturally at a rate of 6–14 cycles per minute.

E. Reciprocal Tension

Once Will Sutherland had determined that the bones of the skull move, he began to contemplate how the separate movements are integrated and from where the motion originates. After much intense study and a thorough review of known concepts, he developed the idea that the dural membranes integrate bony motion. The origin of it all, he theorized is the Breath of Life.

Deciding to create an appropriate name for this integrating function of the dural membranes, he coined the term "reciprocal tension membrane" (RTM). His theory went like this: If all the bones move at once, sometimes cycling in opposing directions, and if the dura unifies them, then the dura must hold a tension for reciprocal action.

Guy wire–like arrangements of dura, crisscrossing through the brain case, offer the means for this reciprocating activity. Dura also holds together all the bones of the cranial base and the vault in a generally spherical configuration. These dural membranes, suspended between the bones and attached to them, are continuous with each other, forming a unit of function.

Sutherland compared the RTM to the wires between two telephone poles; if one pole leans, the next one is pulled by the wires in the same direction by the same distance and at the same time. The arrangement between the falx cerebri and the tentorium cerebelli mimics these mechanics but is more complex. The membranes allow the skull to change its shape but not its volume in cycles of motion. In inhalation, the tentorium and falx cerebri draw in one direction. In exhalation, they reverse their direction.

Sutherland realized from his study of the beveling of the sutures and from palpating his own cranium that the three Cartesian axes change at the same time: (1) in the vertical dimension the base of the skull elevates and the vertex descends, (2) in the anteroposterior dimension the fronto-occipital length decreases, and (3) in the horizontal dimension the bitemporal length widens. Then, the reverse action occurs, creating cycles of motion of inhalation and exhalation. The falx cerebri and tentorium cerebelli, specializations of the dura, coordinate all of this.

Coordinating the specific, cyclical motion of the bones, the membranes also move in a definite manner. Studies of the orientation of the fibers in the falx cerebri and tentorium reveal the direction of the inherent tension that exists within the membranes in the living, thus implying their direction of motion.[50]

In inhalation, the ridgepole of the tentorium cerebelli (the straight sinus) descends and advances anteriorly allowing the sickles of the tent to spread laterally.[51] Simultaneously, the temporal bones slide anteriorly while their squama rock laterally, effectively widening the vault. The falx cerebri similarly descends, moving the vertex in the same direction. It simultaneously draws the mid part (metopic suture) of the frontal bones posteriorly and the occipital squama anteriorly, effectively shortening the anteroposterior diameter of the calvarium. So, we can see the reciprocal action of the membranes in which the tentorium allows for widening, while the falx cerebri pulls the superior, anterior, and posterior aspects of the skull closer to each other. The reverse action occurs in the exhalation phase. (This explanation is simplified; for a complete explanation, please refer to Magoun 1976).

It is along the straight sinus where a moving point of function serves as the fulcrum for all of this bony and membranous activity. *Webster's Third New International Dictionary* defines a "fulcrum" as a mechanical point of stillness around which a lever turns and from which it gains its power. This particular fulcrum, Sutherland said, is (1) *automatic*, an independent and spontaneous mechanical operation; (2) *shifting*, along the length of the straight sinus as changes in tension demand; and (3) *suspended*, within this membrane system. Sutherland's students honored him, years later, by naming this fulcrum along the straight sinus "Sutherland's Fulcrum."

In inhalation, the fulcrum exists in one location along the straight sinus and, in exhalation, in another. As tension changes within the three sickles (the falx cerebri and the two leaves of the tentorium) the position of the fulcrum changes. Even though the shifting fulcrum moves along the straight sinus and the suspended straight sinus itself moves, nevertheless, the fulcrum retains its integrity and its functional power.

Evidence that the dura does indeed integrate the motion of the skull comes from Sutherland's sensitive self-experimentation and from daily clinical work by many practitioners of osteopathy in the cranial field (OCF). This cyclical bony and membranous motion of the skull changes the shape of the skull, not its volume. We will see later that the relative volumes of the skull's contents; that is, blood, cerebrospinal fluid (CSF), and brain, change with pulse pressure and with the inhalation and exhalation phases of the primary respiratory mechanism, but the total volume of the skull remains relatively constant. The important point is that a change in shape without a change in volume depends on the reciprocal tension of the coordinating membranes, the falx cerebri and tentorium cerebelli.

F. Tensegrity

Sutherland independently described something that today is termed "tensegrity."[52] Buckminster Fuller, an architect and philosopher, coined this term to describe the self-supporting nature of the geodesic dome that one of his students designed, combining the words "tensional" and "integrity." "Fuller defined tensegrity as a structural system composed of *discontinuous compression* elements connected by *continuous tension*

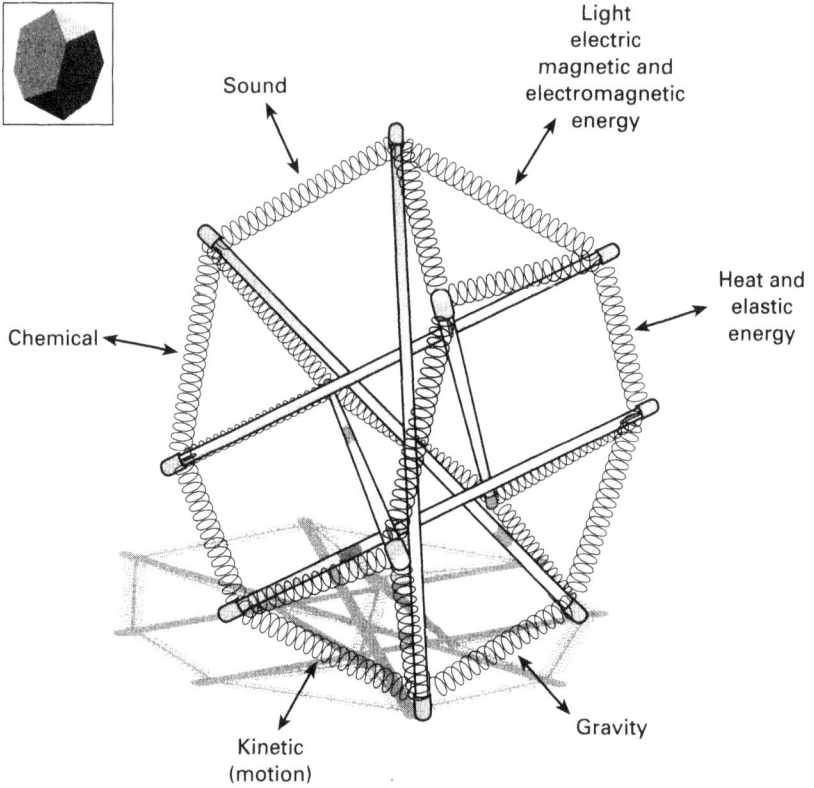

The tensegrity model of Buckminster Fuller is drawn with the "tendons" represented as coils . . . each of the coils has the capability of converting energy from one form to another. Because living tissue is an elastic tensegrous semiconducting continuum, any form of energy can be readily absorbed and conducted from one area to another.

3.4 Tensegrity model. (Reproduced from Oschman JL (2000). *Energy Medicine.* New York: Churchill Livingstone. Fig. 15.8, p. 237. Reprinted with permission from Elsevier Inc.)

cables, which forms a stable structure that can interact in a dynamic fashion."[53]

The simplest example of a tensegrity structure is composed of several incompressible struts that do not touch each other but that are held suspended by a crisscrossing piece of tense string anchoring the ends of the struts. This structure is dynamic—able to fold, twist, and bend—but it retains its integrity and its ability to return to its original shape. Another tensegrity structure is the bicycle wheel. In this structure, the compression elements are the hub and the rim, while the tightened spokes are the tension elements. They provide the means by which forces may be transmitted from the ground to the rider and back again. The spokes hold the rim and hub in a stable but dynamic relationship, sending forces of compression and tension along triangulating straight lines to maintain structural integrity. The triangulation and the tension of the spokes offer a very stable and strong arrangement even though each individual spoke, when disconnected from the unifying tensegrity structure, is weak and can be easily bent.

In the skull, the bones serve as the compression elements and the membranes as the tension cables. Tension in the membranes, as in the spokes of the bicycle wheel, offers a strong, dynamic, and stable structure. The three sickles within the calvarium offer a triangular arrangement in which forces can reciprocate, allowing the calvarium to change its shape but not its volume.

In pathological situations in which trauma has changed the healthy structural and functional relationships, the membranes shift to accommodate the new conformation. For example, Sutherland's Fulcrum may be drawn to the side of increased tension where trauma has induced a restriction of motion. The restoration of positional and functional symmetry is a goal of treatment.

The sacrum, as an example of an element of tensegrity, is relatively stationary, like the hub of a bicycle wheel, within the constant dynamic tension of a system of ligaments, suspending it within the pelvis. In health, the lengths of the ligaments remain practically constant like the spokes of the bicycle wheel, allowing a dynamic balance. If the sacrum moves, other components, which are related to it through ligaments of constant length, will move with the sacrum in "tension-coupled patterns of motion."[54]

These tension-coupled patterns of motion are akin to motion that Sutherland described using the term "nonextensible link."[55] A nonextensible link describes a coordinated, mechanical motion across more than one joint, like the motion of a series of links in a chain. The bones of the skull are linked in such a manner by the dura. They move in a coordinated, dynamic fashion, as a unit, just like the parts of the pelvis all move together. The reciprocal tension membrane operates as one unit, from crown to sacrum, across many joints in the spine and skull.

Curiously, tensegrity does not rely on contractile elements, whereas movement within muscles requires the expenditure of ATP for the ratcheting activity of actin and myosin. However, the sacrum and cranium move without any expenditure of energy within themselves or any muscular action anywhere. Likewise, Sutherland's reciprocal tension membrane is conspicuously missing any contractile fibers. Motions of the bones and membranes are involuntary within the primary respiratory mechanism, just as they are with pulmonary respiration. The sacrum is suspended by an array of ligaments, allowing it to move within the confines of the sacroiliac and lumbosacral joints.

So, the question arises in our minds, as it did in Will Sutherland's, "From where does this cyclical motion originate?" If the sutures demonstrate obvious evidence of the regular activity of the skull bones, and dural membranes integrate that motion without any muscle contraction, how can this palpable motion be explained? Sutherland discovered a clue in a physiology book. He read that the floor of the fourth ventricle contains all the physiological control centers for the body. His mind raced to discover a means by which he could explore the relationship of the fourth ventricle to this motion that resembles involuntary respiration.

G. Compression of the Fourth Ventricle

Sutherland's wife, Adah, discovered him coming out of the back room in his office, "His color was unnatural, his appearance feverish, and his manner disturbingly preoccupied" (Sutherland A, 40). He had been experimenting on himself again. But this time, it would accomplish something that would open up a whole new world, beyond Will Sutherland's already expanded reality.

He had fashioned a split, wooden salad bowl with padding and straps to create a device much like the headrest in a dental chair. This headrest also had straps by which Sutherland could control the tension between the two supports for the back of his head. He had figured out a way to affect the fourth ventricle through his occiput.

He reported to Adah that he had compressed his occiput long enough that he had nearly become unconscious, but he was still able to release the pressure. Then, he felt the most amazing things. " 'A sensation of warmth followed,' he explained. 'And also a remarkable movement of fluid, up and down the spinal column, throughout the ventricles, and surrounding the brain.' His physical experience he summed up in one word: 'Fantastic!'

"During this experiment two surprises had occurred. One seemed to be a *fluctuant* movement of the cerebrospinal fluid as opposed to the orthodox belief that the movement is circulatory. 'That certainly has to be investigated,' he declared. Of the other surprise he exclaimed, 'Believe it or not, there also was a movement of my sacrum! What are we getting into? Is there no end to this?' " (Sutherland A, 40) Sutherland repeated this experiment several times, and each time the sensations were verified. What was the mechanical principle relating the cranium and the sacrum? He felt the concept of the RTM might explain the connection.

Sutherland tested and retested these findings before integrating them into his developing model. He eventually theorized that the pulsation of the CSF determines the motion of the skull and sacrum, and that the pulsation could be used diagnostically and therapeutically. Later, he taught manual maneuvers to direct the tide, as he came to call the palpable fluid fluctuation. We will investigate the tide and its part in the primary respiratory mechanism presently, but first we continue with the story of the membranes and bones.

H. Cranium and Sacrum

Sutherland's next self-experimentation involved his sacrum. He intended to determine the relationship between the cranium and the sacrum. He placed under his supine frame a small hard leather pad at the base of his sacrum to throw it into extreme extension, that is, base anterior.* With this pressure applied to the sacral base, he felt a curious restriction of the CSF and a "dull, heavy sensation" in the cranium. Sutherland used his discovery of the effects of respiratory extension on the sacrum to aid in the treatment of mental illness, including postpartum depression.

Others have satisfactorily proved that a mechanical relationship exists between the cranium and the sacrum without the presence of any contractile elements. Retzlaff and colleagues (1975)[56] demonstrated the relationship between motion in the parietal bones and of the sacrum. They manipulated the sacrum and induced motion in the parietal bones of the squirrel monkey. Electrodes measuring capacitance across sutures recorded the motion of the parietals. Hundreds of clinicians have repeatedly rediscovered that such a relationship not only exists but also is fundamental to the health of their patients.

––––––––––

* This position "extension," with the base anterior, is called flexion in standard biomechanical nomenclature, but Sutherland was working with a respiratory motion. As opposed to ilio-sacral motion of biomechanics, respiratory motion of the sacrum occurs around a fulcrum at the second sacral segment, the only segment where the SI joint reverses its bevel to posterior convergence. The remainder of the joint, displaying anterior convergence, determines the postural motion of the sacrum.

1. Core Link

Referring to the RTM, the sacrum and the cranium are related in motion through what Sutherland called the "core link." He said that the RTM exhibits another pole of attachment beside the ones in the cranium. This is the inferior pole at the second sacral segment. The dura continues from its firm attachment at the foramen magnum, the dens, and body of C-2, and sometimes C-3, loosely attached from there until it reaches another firm attachment at the second sacral segment (with lesser attachments that permit gliding at various lumbar vertebrae). Thus, the cranial base and the sacrum are mechanically related.

2. Nonextensible Link

Referring to the idea of the nonextensible link, the cranial bowl and the pelvic bowl, as distinct from the occiput and sacrum, also demonstrate a mechanical relationship. The connective tissues act as nonextensible links to integrate the motions of these two cavities. In the cranial bowl dura serves this function, and in the pelvic bowl the periosteum, ligaments, and fascia do the same.

The nonextensible links attach firmly to the bones, creating a lining for the bowl and binding the parts into unitary action. The core link relates the two bowls centrally, but many other fascial relationships exist outside the coverings of the central nervous system. Thus, the two bowls operate synchronously in health.

In disease, they can also collude to disturb the normal balance in one bowl if the other is distorted. For example, if we find a temporal bone in a distorted position or pattern of motion, we should also look to see if the ipsilateral pelvic bone is affected similarly. Likewise, we should look for the causes of tinnitus or vertigo in the pelvis, or we may find a related dysfunction in a temporal bone for hip pain.

I. Strain Patterns

In Sutherland's next experiment, he attempted to create in his own cranium an extension head to see what the effects would be in his sacrum. An extension head is long and narrow. Sutherland's head was naturally wide and flat. As lateral compression was applied, his eyesight changed and the orbits were seen to narrow via a handheld mirror. (This finding has been useful in helping to prescribe lenses for vision.) As his vision changed, Sutherland became acutely aware of the central and important role of the sphenoid bone in these and other matters.

He began defining the skull shapes that he visually recognized in people on the street, relating these observations to positions of the sphenoid bone. He astutely observed that an asymmetrically widened and receding orbit, an elevated pinna of the ear, and a sloping forehead to be manifestations of some unspoken trauma. He developed the diagnoses of flexion, extension, torsion, and side-bending rotation patterns, and he defined them according to the relative positions of the base of sphenoid and occipital bones. In 1951, in Magoun's *Osteopathy in the Cranial Field*, he added vertical and lateral strains, intraosseous strains, and compression to the list of lesion patterns of the cranial base (Magoun 1951, 95).

Self-experimentation proceeded with Sutherland producing various strain patterns. To assure his worried wife, Will said, "I am doing this because there is some reason why I must. It has been so the entire way and this is but one more step. I have been taken care of and I know that protection will continue. Amazing things are opening up. I haven't been brought this far only to be let down. There is no need for fear or doubt" (Sutherland A, 54).

His wife commented, "Among his own experiences following production of self-imposed strain, nasal sinuses that had always behaved as they should flared up. Vision, too, varied with the restrictive tests. Concentration, which was outstanding, was noticeably disturbed. Headaches, almost unknown to him as a personal experience, often were nagging and intense. Occasionally, and this was most unnatural, brusqueness and irritability were almost intimidating, and he was strangely remote. What a way to gain knowledge! . . . Others benefit because Dr. Sutherland dared. Had his spadework been shallow, and had the root growth been fostered by guesses, shortcuts, hearsay, and unscientific reasoning, results could not have been so productive, and there would be justification for doubting the validity of his conclusions" (Sutherland A, 57).

Because it is based on *knowledge* and not just *information*, Sutherland's work is validated. Whatever information he gained, Sutherland verified it with knowledge through self-experimentation. His knowledge was based on personal, repeated experience that cannot be denied. Most scientific endeavors justify their conclusions through experiments that separate the observer from the results by the use of some measuring device. Sutherland needed no measuring devices. His experience was direct, directly demonstrating to his senses the function of his own structures. Further, he gained knowledge from another source, contemplation.

J. Visions

Sutherland "privately enjoyed a succinct observation made by Dr. Still: 'Some of us do not have to go to sleep to see visions' " (Sutherland A, 85). "Each day, and this was frequent, he [Sutherland] turned to what he alluded to as 'pause-rest' periods; periods of silence with no outward evidence of activity. This was done with utmost simplicity and naturalness. From these contemplative oases there came some of his most productive reasoning and results. It is why he said with entire sincerity, *'This cranial thought is not mine.'* He liked the phrase[s] 'listening to silence,' . . . 'be still and know,' and 'closer is He than breathing'" (Sutherland A, 65–66; italics added).

Similarly, Still said,

> I do not claim to be the author of this science of Osteopathy. No human hand framed its law; I ask no greater honor than to have discovered it.[57]

Like his predecessor, Drew Still, Will Sutherland accessed the spiritual realm via contemplation to retrieve the knowledge that he passed on to us. Still and Sutherland showed us, as Einstein intimated, that much scientific endeavor generates from spirit. Einstein told of his dreams and thought experiments that preceded his great mathematical discoveries. He "spoke of a 'cosmic religious feeling' that inspired his reflections on the order and harmony of nature . . . Physicists, Brian Josephson and David Bohm believe that regular mystical insights achieved by quiet meditative practices can be a useful guide in the formulation of scientific theories."[58] Still observed that in addition to the traditional five neurological senses, there are "about five hundred other kind of senses on top of them" (Still 1908, 346). Sutherland and Still demonstrated for us how to be fully human, to tap the unseen nature inherent in us all. Knowledge and truth are manifestations of spirit.

Today, our efforts in medicine must include the art of being human, not the science alone. For any medicine, osteopathic or not, to advance toward the expectations that humanity holds for it and to be included in the twenty-first-century paradigm, it must embrace principles of spirit. David Hawkins said, "Medicine had forgotten that it was an *art*, and that science was merely a tool of that art."[59] Osteopathic medicine beautifully combines art and science.

K. Inherent Motility and Fluid Fluctuation

Sutherland invited us to visualize with him the active mechanics of the neural tissue of the brain and the spinal cord.[60] He theorized that, in the inhalation phase, the central nervous system contracts on itself much like an earthworm. Sutherland said, "Swedenborg, 200 years ago, said there is movement of the brain. Have we anything new? No" (Sutherland 1998, 164).

In the embryo, beyond the anterior end of the neural tube (*lamina terminalis*, in the adult), two large expansions develop to form the cerebral hemispheres. Because the embryonic precursors to the membranes and bones of the vault surround these huge appendages as they form, they are forced in their development to curl into two ram's-horn configurations. Therefore, in the adult, the cerebral hemispheres exhibit a motion that resembles a coiling and an uncoiling (Sutherland 1998, 190). With each respiratory cycle, these motions recapitulate the growth and development of the cerebral hemispheres. The hemispheres descend and widen while the diencephalon, brain stem, and spinal cord draw cephalad during inhalation. In exhalation, the opposite motions occur.

The interior canal of the neural tube develops in the adult into the central canal of the spinal cord and the ventricular system of the brain. Conventional belief holds that most of the CSF is produced by the choroid plexuses that are located within the four ventricles of the brain. According to Sutherland, the choroid plexuses perform an additional function—an interchange between the blood and the CSF. This interchange presents an opportunity for the distribution of the "drugs" manufactured in the brain, as Still said, in "God's drugstore" (in Sutherland 1990, 63).[61]

> Believing that a loving, intelligent Maker of man had deposited in his body in some place or throughout the whole system drugs in abundance to cure all infirmities, . . . they can be administered by adjusting

the body in such a manner that the remedies may naturally associate themselves together . . . God or nature is the only doctor whom man should respect. Man should study and use the drugs compounded in his own body. (Still 1908, 88–89)

Sutherland described how the ventricles actively participate in the motion of the CNS. During the inhalation phase of primary respiration, the ependyma, which lines the ventricles, and the pia mater, which covers the exterior of the brain, approximate. Because of the inherent contractile activity of the glial cells, it is theorized that they are responsible for this squeezing action of the brain, much like a sponge. The contractile activity has been proven *in vitro*,[61a] but research still needs to be performed to relate the glial cells to the inherent motion of the CNS.

Sutherland theorized that during the inhalation phase, the volumes of the fluid-containing compartments expand, both within the ventricles (in the interior of the brain) and within the subarachnoid space (on the exterior of the brain). The third ventricle widens from a slit into a V-shape, and its roof lengthens and flattens, stretching out the choroid plexus. Furthermore, the floor of the third ventricle elevates, drawing up the infundibulum and pituitary body. Sutherland said that the pituitary is firmly retained within the sella turcica by the tympanum sellae, a covering over the top of the sella made by a specialization of the dura. The retention of the hypophysis within the sella functions to integrate the motion of the CNS with its container, the dura and bones.

Additional information comes from the intensive and thorough studies of another osteopathic researcher, Charlotte Weaver, DO,[62–65] a contemporary of Sutherland. Still charged Weaver, one of his most promising students, to explore the relationship of osteopathic principles to the head. Weaver spent the remainder of her life studying skulls and their relationship to embryology and the development of the CNS and to pathology.

Weaver discovered that the posterior pituitary (of neural origin) is firmly attached to the floor of the sella turcica. Her detailed studies of fetal, infant, and adult skulls indicated that, in the embryo, the notochord extends forward from the developing spine, through the base of the occipital and sphenoid bones, and into the floor of the sella turcica, terminating in the tissue that becomes the posterior pituitary, the neurohypophysis. This continuity of structure predicts a continuity of function.

Whether we decide that it is via the tympanum sellae, as Sutherland theorized, or via the continuity of the neurohypophysis with the floor of the sella, as Weaver theorized, we have an explanation for the observation by pathologists that the pituitary tends to remain adherent in the skull after the brain is extracted at autopsy. This observation depends on the strength of the tissues of the neural stalk being weaker than the remnants of the notochord.

We might ask ourselves, as Will Sutherland asked himself, "What is the function of this structural adherence to the sella turcica?" We can theorize that such a firm attachment functions to lift the sella turcica as the brain contracts in inhalation. Therefore, as the floor of the third ventricle elevates, it draws the sella turcica superiorly by traction through the infundibulum. The sella occupies the posterior aspect of the body of the basisphenoid. As the sella elevates, it tips the front of the sphenoid body into a nosedive. This motion is consistent with that which Sutherland espoused.

Weaver's information adds a stronger level of evidence, allowing us to comprehend how the brain, membrane, and bony components of the primary respiratory mechanism integrate their motions. The tympanum sellae performs an important function as well, whether or not it participates in the bony motion. It helps to pump the pituitary body as the infundibulum compresses the bulging adenohypophysis and neurohypophysis up against this tense dural covering. Without this activity, hormone delivery to the rest of the organism could be wanting.

In a similar fashion, the lateral ventricles elevate on their posterior aspects within the coiling cerebral hemispheres, widening the calvarium. In exhalation, they fold down, allowing the skull to narrow, while the floor of the third ventricle descends, releasing the infundibulum and the basisphenoid inferiorly (Sutherland 1998, 192). This pumping facilitates the exchange of contents between the ventricles and the blood of the choroid plexuses as their shapes lengthen and shorten.

Still referred to the brain as a dynamo, implying that its motion generates an electrical charge that is transmitted by the nerves to drive the whole system. Likewise, Sutherland explained that the brain has inherent motion and that the potency of the CSF is partly electrochemical, acquired through its intimate contact with the brain. As early as 1971, neurologists at Queen's University, in Kingston, Ontario, Canada, described brain motion resembling Traube-Hering waves.[66] (Traube, Hering, and Mayer discovered cyclic variations in the pulse pressure of cannulated dog carotid arteries in the mid- and late 1800s; see Chapter Four for more on Traube and Hering.)

Radiographic studies have recently shown that the brain has dynamo-like activity. These investigators were not looking for motions in the brain that are slower than vascular pulsations, but their results nevertheless confirm that the diencephalon, brain stem and cerebellum, as Still declared one hundred years earlier, pump up and down, driving brain motion and CSF fluctuations.[67] (More on this topic appears in the next chapter.)

L. Sutherland Digs On

In speaking of his experiences, Sutherland had said, "I would be fearful of becoming an inmate of one of our many [mental] institutions if I confided this to fellow colleagues" (Sutherland A, 52). In spite of this fear, he continued to move forward. Will Sutherland warned his wife that "If the time did come when his cranial conclusions should be made known, there would be those within the profession who would be skeptical, who might attach uncomplimentary labels, and that the way would not be soft. It did not occur to him that dissenters within his profession would resort to harsh condemnation of his contribution without first investigating it. Or be so uncharitable as to employ offensive personal attacks. But that has been the lamentable experience of many an intrepid innovator" (Sutherland A, 52). Just as Still did before him, Sutherland valued the truth that he was uncovering more than his personal reputation.

At first, Sutherland ventured to share his new knowledge with his family, treating them. Then he added a few carefully selected patients to the circle. Treatment results proved favorable, and he soon had referrals from patients. His success in treating migraines, sinusitis, strabismus, asthma, bronchitis, and mental illness assured him that he must share this osteopathic contribution with his colleagues. So, in 1929, he vowed to do so, despite the lack of substantiation from accepted scientific sources. He knew that the clinical benefits outweighed any biased or intolerant reaction he might receive from others. He also knew that the scientific substantiation would come.

M. The Breath of Life

Sutherland concluded that the fluctuation of the fluid was fundamental to the primary respiratory mechanism.[68] The motion of the brain, its ventricles, and the subarachnoid space are integral to the fluctuation of the fluid. He determined that the motion of the other components, the bones and membranes, are secondary to the fluid dynamics. These other components passively accommodate the inherent, active motion of the brain and the potent fluctuation of the fluid. Bones and membranes have mobility; the brain has motility; and the fluid has potency.

Sutherland quoted Still, who said,

> The cerebrospinal fluid is the highest known element that is contained in the human body.[69]

Sutherland referred to the highest known element as the Breath of Life. From original cause, the stillness of the Breath of Life, a motion derives. This vital force, an effect of the Breath of Life, manifests as an active, generative behavior in the CSF. The CSF activates the whole central nervous system and its covering: neurons, glial cells, meninges, skull, spine, and sacrum. What is the origin of this vital action? Sutherland implied that the origin was unknown and that it was not necessary to understand it in order to apply it usefully for healing. He said that the potency of the CSF has several identifiable characteristics.

1. Electrochemical Potency

First there is an electrochemical property. Because the cerebral hemispheres coil and uncoil, they resemble a dynamo. Through this dynamo-like activity, the brain develops a polarity and the CSF acquires an electrical charge.

Still wrote in his *Autobiography*,

> your brain with its two lobes [is] an electric battery. When the cerebellum sets this dynamo in motion, oxygen is carried through the system and vitalizes the blood, the abdomen, the eye, and the entire man. Nature put this battery in you to keep the blood healthy and salts it with oxygen. (Still 1908, 233)

Still went further to explain that electricity is the element that is vital for the action of oxygen in the body. Health requires the "life-giving current," which is natural and which he called "God's method," whereas intrusions using artificial drugs he called "uncertain."

Think of yourself as an electric battery. Electricity seems to have the power to explode or distribute oxygen, from which we receive the vitalizing benefits. When it plays freely through your system, you feel well. Shut it off in one place and congestion results, in this case a medical doctor, by dosing you with drugs, would increase this congestion until it resulted in decay. He is like the Frenchman who lets his duck rot that it may boil the sooner. Not so with an Osteopath. He removes the obstruction, lets the *life-giving current* have full play, and the man is restored to health. The one is man's way and is uncertain, the other is God's method and is infallible. Choose this day whom you will serve. (Still 1908, 235; italics added)

Still also wrote,

All must have, and cannot act without the highest known order of force (electricity), which submits to the voluntary and involuntary commands of life and mind, by which worlds are driven and beings move. (Still 1908, 195)

We can infer from these words that Still understood that the highest known element directs the highest known order of force, electricity or, perhaps, that Still felt electricity and the highest known element were one and the same.

Sutherland said, "I call your attention to the water, the clear water, in the battery of your car. You have chemicals in that water, material chemicals. But you cannot see the invisible element, the electrical 'juice' that comes from that water, that passes along the wire that runs to the motor of your car. That is the *potency*, the power, that comes from the battery" (Sutherland 1990, 32; italics added).

Sutherland is quoted as saying, "Our knowledge is like that of the electrician who merely *knows* that the potent current, or M-element* [mutual inductance], is present and that he is learning *how to utilize its force*. We, too, merely *know* that the cerebrospinal fluid is present and contains the 'highest known element' and that we are learning, through the cranial concept, *how to utilize its force* in behalf of the ills of mankind" (Sutherland 1998, 273; italics in original).

Sutherland also referred to a coaxial cable to create a mental image for his students. The cable can carry many messages simultaneously for great distances without loss of strength. Within a coaxial cable are many copper tubes that are insulated from each other. Then, inside each tube is a wire that is insulated from the copper tube. A potential exists within this system that allows its extraordinary function. Between the wire and the tube is information.

Sutherland hypothesized that within a nerve trunk the highest known element is formed like the information is formed within the potential of the coaxial cable. Many messages are carried simultaneously, needing only the right receiver to be tuned to the correct frequency for the proper information. This is not the "usual way that messages are carried by nerve fibers" (Sutherland 1990, 32–33). Sutherland compared the nerves of the infundibulum to a coaxial cable. Nerves throughout the body are constructed in a similar fashion, the perineurium being compared to the space between the copper tube and the copper wire in the coaxial cable. Information can be carried in this space.

2. Potency through Transmutation

Sutherland said, "Visualize that 'something' in the cerebrospinal fluid that has a transmutation in the nerve cells or tracts, or in a 'copper tube.' It doesn't flow along the nerve fibers as though they were wires. It is a change in form, if you wish. It doesn't run something. That something

---

* "M-element" is an electrical term meaning mutual inductance. A varying electric current produces a varying magnetic field that induces voltages in the same circuit or in a nearby circuit.

is in the tubes" (Sutherland 1990, 33).

Sutherland explained that the "highest known element, the cerebrospinal fluid, the element that is thought by the cranial concept to provide nourishment to the brain cells with consequent *transmutation* of the element throughout nerve fiber to terminal. Perhaps this transmutation is the nerve force to which Dr. Still referred" (Sutherland 1998, 215; italics in original).

Sutherland brought to our attention the activity within a lymph node as an example of transmutation. Before infected lymph can be delivered back to the bloodstream, it must be changed so the infection will not affect the rest of the organism. A transmutation—a change into another nature, substance, form, or condition—occurs in the lymph node.

Sutherland taught that at the still point that comes when compressing the fourth ventricle, the highest known element causes a transmutation. There is an interchange among all the fluids of the body, and a change, or transmutation, occurs in that fluid. Sutherland said, "It is not an outflow over the nerves, although the change follows along to the area where the terminals of the peripheral nervous system dwell with the lymphatics. The change is in the constituents, or elements, through transmutation. This is quite different from transmission, or outflow. I want you to see that 'highest known element' in the human body going out in that transmutation from the nerve cell along the fibers to the terminals. Then, perhaps, you will grasp more clearly what Dr. Still meant when he said that the lymphatics consume more of the waters of the brain than the entire viscera" (Sutherland 1990, 176).

3. Intelligence of the Tide

Learning to work with the potency of the CSF has profound effects. "In using the direction of the Tide for correction, for treatment, you use the same direction process that you used for diagnosis . . . If you did nothing other than direct that Tide, there would be, in time, a correction of the lesion" (Sutherland 1990, 176–177).

Still wrote,

> **God's intelligence is immeasurable, and there is much evidence that knowledge is imparted to the corpuscle of the blood before it does its work. (Still 1908, 185)**

Sutherland often referred to the Intelligence (he capitalized the word) of the tide. According to Sutherland, one has greater success with treatment if one engages the unerring potency or unerring Intelligence from within, instead of using blind force from without.

In diagnosis, if one feels the tide rebound from the area opposite from where he or she is directing it, then one knows there is an obstruction in that place. "The diagnostic rebound is specific. You do not even have to test for the pattern of mobility at the sphenobasilar junction. The Tide will tell you. It is uncanny" (Sutherland 1990, 167).

"How do I direct the Tide? This is even more uncanny. You would expect the flow to go directly to some point, but it doesn't. I am not going to tell you how it gets there because I don't know, but it gets there . . . This Tide is directed gently by the touch of a finger" (Sutherland 1990, 168). "Visualize a potency, an intelligent potency, that is more intelligent than your own human mentality . . . You will have observed its potency and also its Intelligence, spelled with a capital *I*. It is something you can depend upon to do the work for you. In other words, don't try to drive the mechanism through any external force. Rely upon the Tide" (Sutherland 1990, 14).

4. Liquid Light

Sutherland explained that the primary respiratory mechanism manifests because the Breath of Life permeates the body like "sheet lightning illuminates a cloud" (Sutherland 1998, 291). He invited us to visualize with him how light passes through glass; glass is a fluid made of sand, and sand comes from solid rock. He asked us to visualize the space between the elements of the rock and to compare that to the space between the material substances of the body (Sutherland 1998, 295–296).

He suggested that the "highest known element" is invisible but may be illustrated in the potency that lights up x-ray film. (Sutherland 1998, 291). The Breath of Life, he said, is liquid light; it exists in the fluid between the fibers, as Swedenborg intimated two hundred years before Sutherland. Swedenborg said that the love and wisdom of God flows from the heavenly sun and invests itself with the material of the earth to create the form of the body and to move it (see Chapter Two, Section II.A: "Emmanuel Swedenborg"). Similarly, Dante said, "The love of God, unutterable and perfect, flows into a pure soul the way that light rushes into a transparent object."

James Jealous, DO, followed Sutherland's line of thinking and expressed for us the reality of the physical human organism existing in a sea of energy, the Love of God. Jealous compared this reality to Rachel Carson's message in her book, *The Sea Around Us* by saying, "The sea around us is more than a Deep Silence. Its presence is Love."[70] The Love of God is present everywhere, preexisting, generating, and permeating everything. Our physical forms exist in this sea, differentiating from it only by having managed to reduce the vibration of its material constituents as they manifest.

Sutherland said, "Where is that cerebrospinal fluid? Is it only in my body? No. It is in each and every one of your bodies. There is an ocean of cerebrospinal fluid in this room. Here is a *fluid within a fluid*. There is a *fluid within a fluid*. The Breath of Life is within each. You know something about shortwave, don't you? It goes from one pole to another. It passes right through an individual" (Sutherland 1990, 169). "Another uncanny event has happened. While balancing the cranial membranous articular mechanism, another person can sit back a ways and direct the Tide to a foot without touching the foot. I know this sounds fantastic, but I am telling you these facts from experience. Also, I have heard reports from others who have tried it out" (Sutherland 1990, 168).

N. X-Ray Vision

Sutherland said, "That is the picture I want you to see as the 'highest known element' in the cerebrospinal fluid. *An invisible element.* Something that may be illustrated in the potency that lights up the film in taking an x-ray picture. Something you do not see, but it lights up the x-ray film. It is not visible. You merely see the spark from the positive and negative poles—it jumps from one pole to the other. But you do not see the real element because you are the man formed from the earth and walking about utilizing this breath of air. If you recognized the real element, the Breath of Life in the fluctuation of the cerebrospinal fluid, I think you would begin to come closer to the success of Dr. Still in his knowledge of the human body. He had not only the material knowledge through his dissections etcetera of those early days but also his experience as an Army surgeon, the practical clinical experience. Besides that, he recognized a highest known element in the cerebrospinal fluid. You might say he was like the x-ray; he could look right through you and see things, and tell you things, without even putting his hands upon your body. I have seen him do that! Time and time again. When some of the early teachers had a clinic up before the class, hunting for the lesion, in would come the Old Doctor from the rear, 'Here's your lesion.' How did he do it?" (Sutherland 1998, 291).

Students of Sutherland speak privately of his skill in recognizing structural distortions from a distance, without palpating. This skill is common among other practitioners since Still and Sutherland, some of whom are practicing as this book is written. It is nothing more than the simple application of natural human abilities that are trained, strengthened, and finely honed. Still referred to this phenomenon as coming from the realm of Mind. Still told a student that the mind should be able to view the body as the x-ray, if one raises the vibration.

Jealous, Danté, and Swedenborg reminded us that the Love of God is the source of physical reality. David Bohm (see Chapter Two, Section II.H) described this originating reality as the implicate order; William Tiller called it the reciprocal space. The ideas of Bohm and Tiller grew out of quantum physics, and, indeed, it is the impact of quantum physics that modern medicine must and will soon integrate. Non-locality and the effects of the mind on matter are quantum effects that Larry Dossey described as principles of Era III medicine (see Chapter Two, Section II.G).

Still and Sutherland were describing these same quantum effects in medicine before quantum mechanics was defined, in the case of Still, or widely understood, in the case of Sutherland. They reiterated for us the human ability to use Mind in the process of healing. In osteopathic treatment, the intention of the physician and patient figure prominently in healing. Still reminded us, while treating patients, to keep in our minds the image of the normal anatomy as the painter keeps the image of the scene or beast that he wishes to represent with his brush.

Osteopathy benefits from having already recognized this quantum reality and from the resultant knowledge of its clinical application. Osteopathic physicians have the opportunity to integrate modern physics and ancient themes by thoroughly applying osteopathic principles from Still and Sutherland; and osteopathic medicine is positioned by its history and perspective to integrate this modern and ancient reality into today's conventional medicine. Integrative medicine can use osteopathic medicine as a template. Era III medicine can rightly emerge from within the principles of osteopathic medicine. Osteopathic medicine could lead this great revolution in medicine by simply practicing and teaching the principles outlined by Still, Sutherland, and their eminent students.

O. Spirit in Osteopathy

Sutherland said, "I have often said that we lost something in oste-opathy that Dr. Still tried to get across. That was the spiritual that he included in the science of osteopathy . . . What came was the concept of osteopathy. What does he say? 'It came as did other truths that came to benefit mankind.' Read his *Research and Practice* and see how many times you can see the reference to his Creator, the Great Architect, et-cetera. He is continually calling your attention to that" (Sutherland 1998, 293).

In 1950, Robert Truhlar, DO, published a book of quotations from Andrew Still that he had collected from osteopathic colleagues around the United States in order to express the "spiritual understanding" of Osteopathy that the older doctors in the profession understood. At the time of its publication, the practicing DOs who were students of Still were coming to the ends of their lives. Truhlar wanted to capture the essence of their collective understanding of Osteopathy that they had acquired directly from Still. In the preface of his book, *Doctor A. T. Still in the Living*, Truhlar characterized their basic understanding of Still's philosophy as "spiritual."[71] Apparently, Truhlar, who was not a student of Still, had realized that the osteopathic profession was losing the focus of its initial, inherited purpose. For the osteopathic philosophy to be transmitted properly, the first generation of Still's students needed to interpret Still's philosophy for those who would succeed them.

Under the difficult circumstances in which the profession began and in which it carried on after the death of its indomitable founder, the lineage of inheritance seemed tenuous. Spirituality, as unpopular a focus as it was for any profession, served only to magnetize further discrimination to a social group that simply wanted acceptance in order to provide the services that its collective membership knew it could provide. Yet tied to this knowledge of professional capability was the pain of nonacceptance and potential demise.

The osteopathic profession then enacted a scenario, which any group that suffers discrimination will invariably enact. It denied its distinctiveness to avoid the pain and its potential demise from nonacceptance. Without the strength and the vision of its founder to sustain it, the profession melded into the sameness of its environment. Spirituality was forsaken as a reason to exist because it threatened existence.

Today, the osteopathic medical profession continues to deal with the effects of intense and unrelenting discrimination without the benefit of its founder to withstand such pressure and to articulate the purpose for the profession's persistence. It was a simple case of Drew Still being ahead of his time. Well, the time has now arrived for his ideas to be accepted, and today's osteopathic physicians can champion them, if we choose to do so.

P. Spirit in Treatment

William Garner Sutherland, DO, rekindled the element of spirit in the philosophy of Osteopathy with his theory of the primary respiratory mechanism. He advanced the spiritual aspect of Osteopathy because the philosophy of A. T. Still had been imprinted on and prepared his mind. "Dr. Still has taken my hand in his and allowed me to feel the lesion as it is being exaggerated and then as the natural agencies pulled the bones back into place" (Sutherland 1998, 160). Sutherland began his research into the spirit of osteopathic philosophy when he made his brilliant observation that the bony skull demonstrates evidence for respiratory motion. Then, with detailed exploration of inanimate skulls, he determined that the dural membranes integrate the motion. And finally, after years of self-experimentation on his living skull and contemplation, he became convinced that the source of the motion is the Breath of Life. The life force as the prime mover fit perfectly with what Still taught him, that biogen, the most primitive example of Matter in Motion, receives its vitality from the Great Architect. Further, in the fully developed organism, the health of the tissues depends on a continual supply of spiritual influence. Still wrote, "All that gives you life and health comes straight from heaven" (Truhlar, 64).

Sutherland merely worked out a mechanism that elucidated Still's general philosophical framework. He pointed to Still's discoveries as the source of his own teaching. He said, like Still did, that he had only discovered natural principles. He did not take credit for original concepts, although this seems too modest. Sutherland's intention was to honor the founder of Osteopathy as the source of his ideas because Still had indeed set the stage for all that Sutherland came to understand. In Still's writing we see that he laid out in embryonic form all of Sutherland's concepts. In fact, if we read between the lines of Still's writings, as Sutherland invited us to do, it is obvious that Still already understood all that Sutherland eventually promulgated.

Sutherland directed his students to "Think Osteopathy" (Sutherland 1998, 293). He said, "In technique we endeavor to follow Dr. Still's methods—that is, getting the point of release with no jerking and then allowing the natural agencies to return the bones to their normal relations and positions. What are the natural agencies? The ligaments, not the muscles, are the natural agencies for this purpose of correcting the relations and positions at joints. Dr. Still's application of the technique is the gentle exaggeration of the lesion that allows the natural agencies to draw the bones back into place . . . We have something more potent than our own forces working always in the patient towards the direction of normal" (Sutherland 1998, 160).

In summary, studying Sutherland is studying Still. Osteopathy's promise lies in the principles espoused by Still and in their evolution by others, including Sutherland. Practicing cranial osteopathy is practicing Osteopathy close to Still. Still wrote, "An intelligent head will soon learn that a soft hand and a gentle move is the hand and the head that get the desired results" (in Truhlar, 64).

III. RECAPITULATION AND LOOKING AHEAD

The reciprocity between Still's Celestial and Terrestrial realms not only describes creation but also characterizes an ongoing influence in the living organism. This reciprocity manifests in the living organism moment by moment as a palpable oscillation, which Sutherland referred to as the Tide. When spirit invests matter, the material substance oscillates with vitality.

A familiar example of an oscillation imposed by an outside source of power is a branch of a tree dipping in the water at the edge of a stream that wiggles back and forth in the passing current. The less vital connective tissues oscillate as the vital fluids impart the life force to them. The Tide in the fluids is the expression of spirit, the Breath of Life. The Breath of Life is in the unseen and the Tide manifests in the visible (palpable) world.

In its most basic palpable function, the Tide cyclically resonates in the fluids and moves the tissue matrix. In its greater functional ramifications, the Tide also creates metabolic activity. As we explore in the next chapter, this metabolic activity is defined in the physiology texts as tissue respiration.

Sutherland named this function well, the primary respiratory mechanism. It is a functional mechanism that manifests from the implicate order into the explicate order, existing in the tissues as something that can be palpated. It is a respiratory metabolic activity that delivers health from the implicate order to the explicate order in the tissues, bringing nutrition to the cell and carrying metabolic wastes away. It comes from that which precedes everything, that which is primary, that is, the Love of God, which exists in the implicate order, manifesting the breath of air in the explicate order. Sutherland's discovery of the primary respiratory mechanism may one day be recognized as a fundamental turning point in the ongoing development of physiology.

The fluctuation of fluid is a mechanism of Health. Health, with a capital *H*, implies an activity, not just a condition, a verb, not a noun. Health originates from, exists in, and permeates the tissues. As Steve

Paulus, DO, stated, "It generates all of the fundamental forces involved with healing. Health is undifferentiated, non-directional, and unorganized. The Health provides the raw material for healing,"[72] like biogen. It maintains the body in a living, functioning, and healthy condition. It emanates as an aspect of the potency of the fluids. The potency of the fluids, as described by Sutherland, is mandatory for life.

Healing happens when diseased tissues that have been cut off from this supply are once again nourished by it. The return to the tissues of the influence of spirit, called healing, is a divine act because it resupplies divinity where it has been deprived but where it belongs. CSF, blood, lymph, and extracellular and intracellular fluids carry this divine nourishment, information, and knowledge from the Mind of God.

At the next level, a healing process, unlike Health, has a distinct direction and purpose. As Still indicated, the Mind of God directs each corpuscle. This direction from the Mind of God comes easily through the vehicle we know as water. In the next chapter, we explore how water is just as unusual as it is common.[73]

Still declared that the brain is a dynamo that produces electricity and that the fluid surrounding it contains the highest known element. Sutherland declared that Still's highest known element in the CSF operates by transmutation throughout the nerves to affect the lymph and the rest of the fluids of the body. He proclaimed that there is an interchange among all the fluids of the body at the still point, when the oscillation is brought down to an idling.

Steve Paulus wrote, "Many Osteopaths do not know that normal function can be perverted in the non-material field, outside of what is termed soma. Lesions do not just occur in bones, muscles, connective tissues, and nerves. We can also utilize a non-material, non-mechanical approach to help restore the organism to a higher level of functioning. The Health, Tides, and other nonmaterial forces of healing can be applied to physical or non-physical lesions/dysfunctions."[74] The space around the physical form becomes as important as the form itself. The

Breath of Life permeates the totality of creation, both the material and the nonmaterial. Mind/emotions exist in the nonmaterial realm of Bohm and Tiller and in the Celestial realm of A. T. Still. An individual heals as distortions of influences from material and nonmaterial sources resolve into symmetry.

On the physical side, treatment using the primary respiratory mechanism relies on the potency of the tide. First, we activate the potency by compressing, disengaging, or balancing the tension in the tissues. Once it has been stimulated into action, we merely observe the effects of the potency by palpation and learn how it decompresses compressions, rebalances tensions, and rediscovers the original. The potency of the fluids unwinds the tissues until it achieves a still point out of which evolves an easy normal oscillation.

At the still point, a transmutation and exchange among all fluid compartments of the body occurs. A transmutation—a change in the constituents, character, or nature of the fluids—is the means by which the potency expresses the new condition of the treated tissues. With the establishment of a normal palpable cycle of fluid fluctuation comes improved joint motion, circulation of blood and lymph, neural and organ function, and metabolic activity. Sutherland called the potency "Intelligent" and "unerring," borrowing the latter term from Still, who referred to the unerring effects of the Mind of God. Sutherland explained these phenomena by referring to the potency as "unexplainable" because it emanates from the unknowable Mind of God.

Despite the unexplained nature of the potency, we know the phenomenon of potency is real because on a purely practical level, many clinicians routinely prove its existence by palpating and working with the phenomenon and demonstrating the efficacy of potency for healing. Further, subjective and objective clinical results confirm changes that occur in patients from the potency of fluids. Patients and clinicians feel, sometimes simultaneously, structural shifts within the body of the patient during treatment. Patients and clinicians observe, through time, changes in patients' symptom patterns and functional ability. Physicians also observe, through time, the alteration of strain patterns that are palpable in patients.

To help explain Sutherland's "unexplainable" nature of potency, we can refer to modern research performed since Sutherland. William Tiller (see Chapter Two, Section II.I) contributed a new vision of reality that helps us understand the workings of the Mind as described by Still and Sutherland. Tiller defined mind as an aspect of the "reciprocal space" in which light travels at the speed of light squared and the influence of mind moves matter. He also reported a phenomenon in which the influence of mind (intention) over time affects the space in which the intention resides to produce an oscillation of various measurable parameters, such as temperature and pH. This phenomenon of the oscillation of measurable parameters in a space conditioned by the influence of mind (intention) may be a general phenomenon and may prove to explain the oscillation of the fluid in the tissues that Sutherland called the tide.

We could consider the Greater Mind to occupy the space around the physical body and to interpenetrate it. The influence of Mind as described by Danté, Swedenborg, the Taoists, Sheldrake, and Still all fit with this modeling. Sutherland simply added to these other concepts the practical observation of a fluid oscillation and its potency for healing.

In Tiller's experiments, intention changed the pH and the activity of enzymes. By extrapolation, we may conclude that the intention of the osteopathic physician, in which he or she holds the normal anatomy in mind and simultaneously accesses the potency of the Tide, alters the activity of enzymes in the connective tissues. This could explain the phenomenon that clinicians routinely observe in which the connective tissues refashion themselves when one uses the tide in treatment.

As we investigate in the next chapter, the conformation of the connective tissues depends on their charge and shape. The potency of the fluids is responsible for the maintenance and/or the alteration—through transformation—of the charge and shape of the connective tissues. The potency of the fluids is a manifestation of the unseen effects of spirit into the realm of the visible. Tiller's observation that intention creates an observable oscillation explains how an influence in the implicate order (Bohm) through holomovement reveals itself in the explicate order. This oscillation generated from mind in a rigorously defined experiment shows the activity of spirit in the observable world.

If the "fascia is the dwelling place of the spirit," according to Still, and if life is found in the "juices between the fibres," according to Swedenborg, then the fascia is the container of spirit and the fluids reveal the activity of spirit. In osteopathic treatment, spirit in the fluid changes its solid container. And spirit delivers health.

Outside the physical, Mind is ever active and able to alter the physical as well as the nonphysical. The healing of the psyche occurs simultaneously with the physical if we realize the inseparability of mental/emotional and physical attributes. Usually, this culture's dualistic paradigm separates in our view of reality these physical and nonphysical aspects, separating their healing as well. If we adopt quantum effects into our understanding of reality and see physical and nonphysical as different aspects of the same thing, they will behave as one, in illness and healing. David Bohm said that meaning links mind and matter like opposite sides of a coin.[75]

A change in pH is a transmutation, that is, a change in form, nature, or substance. Sutherland attributed the potency of the tide with the ability to transmute. Lowering the pH of water by intention, as Tiller accomplished in his experiments, fundamentally changes the constituents of water. It increases the numbers of hydrogen ions. In order to accomplish this task, hydrogen must break chemical bonds with oxygen, liberating oxygen molecules into the water and the surrounding air. The reverse process takes place when the pH is elevated.

With changes in pH come changes in electrochemical conductivity, oxygen tension, and other physiologically important characteristics of the fluid, that is, other aspects of transmutation. Tiller gave us a simple demonstration of the activity of Mind affecting chemistry and physiology. Still declared Mind to be fundamental to Osteopathy; Sutherland developed a practical system to work directly with Mind to benefit patients; and Tiller described a testable framework to show how Mind works.

This early evidence from Tiller's work and from the theories of Bohm, Swedenborg, Sheldrake, and others confirm the declarations of Still and Sutherland that Mind influences material substance. They also point to the manner by which material creation comes into being, something Still referred to frequently in his writings. He said that Mind and Matter reciprocate to produce material form and to move it.

Chaos theory holds that attractors determine outcomes and that minute variations at the beginning of a process have monumental consequences as the process matures over time. Attractors are the organizing principles around which activities and forms coalesce. All of nature behaves as it does because of attractors. Chaos theory uncovered the existence and the effects of attractors as organizing principles of nature, demonstrating through mathematics that what appears to be disorganized or chaotic is only a matter of perception. All of nature has underlying organization on some level, although unfettered choice among infinite possibilities continues to exist. Looking more deeply reveals an organization that comes from the unseen aspect of creation. The unseen aspect of Mind holds patterns or fields that Sheldrake characterized as morphogenic fields. Still described the operation of the unseen as the Celestial realm. These unseen patterns emerge into the explicate order of Bohm as material forms and behaviors.

The meaning of the attractor determines whether a form or activity more or less aligns with health or disease.[76–79] Love produces effects that strengthen the contraction of muscles and the oscillation of the tide, in my personal experience. Hate produces weakness of the same. David Hawkins opened our eyes to this potential. If the meaning of the attractor comes from something close to love or joy, its consequences will be health and success. If it comes from something close to anger or revenge, it will produce an effect that eventually succumbs in sickness or failure. Hawkins wrote, "All the great teachers throughout the history of our species have merely taught one thing, over and over, in whatever language, at whatever time. All have said, simply: Give up weak attractors for strong attractors" (Hawkins 2002, 141). This phenomenon of weakness versus strength of physiological responses to mental/emotional attitudes lies at the heart of sickness and wellness. Research into this field will eventually yield enormous benefits to humankind.

Once created, the living organism needs continual input from Mind to maintain itself. Mind offers the necessary attractors for ongoing function. The influence of Mind comes from the creative impulse, from the individual and from his or her associations. The physician, as an associate of a patient, can serve an important function for that individual.

Because Mind and Matter are one, the normal anatomy of the individual's origin holds great promise for his or her continuation of health. The resumption of the normal shape of the container of the patient is a return to the original creative impulse that emanated from the Love of God. The fluids of the body transport this influence from Mind as health for this ongoing resupply of the tissues. Distorted tissues impede this fluid impulse.

Circulation and oscillation are both required to refresh the needs of the material form. The primary respiratory mechanism intimately nourishes the cellular elements on a local level, distributing individual properties to the cell membranes from the gross supply lines of the arterial blood. The tide-like motion in the extracellular space is necessary to deliver nutrition and to remove waste products from the parenchymal cells. It stands to reason that passive diffusion is not sufficient to provide quantities and types of elements rapidly enough for the voracious needs of the cells. The distance from the nutritive capillary is too far, and the gel-like intervening substance in the extracellular matrix is too daunting. Another active mechanism must breach this functional chasm. That mechanism is the tide, driven by the life force. We investigate some of the details of this further in the next chapter.

Still proposed that biogen, charged with the life force, is the basic unit of life. As Pischinger said, the fundamental structure of life is a triad, composed of the cell, the extracellular space, and the nutrient capillary. The extracellular space, according to Pischinger's model, becomes critical for the maintenance of life. As we explore in the next chapter, the extracellular space threatens the survival of the cell because of its potential to limit the delivery of nutrients and the discharge of wastes. Mechanisms of health that manifest as oscillations assure the survival of cells.

Oscillations are everywhere in cellular physiology. They pick up where circulation ends. Oscillations are like the waves on the beach that resolve the tides of the ocean where they interface with land. Fluids in the body interface with the solid aspects of the organism as oscillations. As we see in the next chapter, oscillations of physiology play a role in determining the pH, delivering oxygen and other nutrients, and polymerizing and depolymerizing the glucoaminoglycans that are wont to create an obstructing gel in the extracellular matrix.

Osteopathic manipulative treatment facilitates these mechanisms of health. Once the alignment of bones, ligaments, and fascia is achieved, neurovascular arrangements and the tide become unimpeded and health is once again available to the tissues. Whatever means the operator uses to deliver health requires a fine understanding of functional anatomy. In the paradigms of Still and Sutherland, as elucidated by the paradigm of quantum mechanics, the osteopathic physician must also understand energetic, nonphysical, and spiritual realities.

4

A NEW VIEW

It is the finite that suffers. The infinite lies stretched in smiling repose.
— RALPH WALDO EMERSON

I. INTRODUCTION

The explorer for truth must first declare his independence of all obligations or brotherhoods of any kind whatsoever. He must be free to think and reason. — A. T. STILL

Woven throughout this book is the intention to enhance and broaden our comprehension of the wisdom of Dr. Still's philosophy. But to reach for more understanding requires that together, the writer and reader of this book must follow Still's example. Like Drew Still, we, as explorers toward an understanding of the construction of the world, must be willing to adopt a new paradigm, to step back from the realm of conventional thinking, and to entertain new ideas or to look at old ones from new perspectives. We must apply new information to old concepts, look at modern physiological and biochemical realities through new eyes, and even peer through Still's eyes with new and greater insight.

As Paul Kimberly, DO, so aptly asserted in his Scott Memorial Lecture,[1] there are no true osteopathic principles, only principles of nature that Still crafted into a very useful and practical approach to patients from which each osteopathic physician might develop his or her own treatments. The essential elements of A. T. Still's philosophy, as I understand them, appear in summary in the Appendix. These elements I have interpreted in the light of his writings and other diverse sources of information, some of which Still did not have available to him.

This chapter elucidates osteopathic phenomena—natural phenomena. I trust this writing encourages and contributes to beneficial discussions regarding the essence of nature, healing, and Osteopathy.

II. SUMMARY OF STILL'S PHILOSOPHY IN A NEW LIGHT

We can analyze material bodies but we have to stop at the life line for more knowledge. — A. T. STILL

To briefly summarize Dr. Still's philosophy using my own terms, two elements combine to create a life form and to move it. Those two elements are spirit and matter, with consciousness directing the process.

The material element requires the life force to vitalize it in the living organism. Without the infusion of spirit (that which is infinite), the material body (that which is finite) could not be characterized as containing life. On the other hand, the container must possess the attributes necessary to receive and accommodate that which spirit imparts, thus creating a material form that exhibits motion—the two requisites of material life. Connective tissues have interesting properties that receive and respond to life's impulse. Indeed, connective tissue is the material vessel of life.

To imbue the material element with the life force, something less fixed than connective tissue must interpose itself between spirit and matter. Water proves to be that substance to perfection. Water conforms to the shape of its container. It carries and transfers energy (information) that spirit provides to stimulate metabolism. In solution, the necessary elements exist to carry on the activities of life.

Water brings together certain minerals, amino acids, and hormones for anabolic functions, literally transforming energy from the ethereal realm into substance in the material realm. Within the medium of a watery bath, catabolic reactions take energy from the ethereal realm to produce adenosine triphosphate (ATP), the currency of energy in the material realm. Thus, water mediates between the implicate order and the explicate order to manifest the activities of life in the physical realm.

Water also participates in the creation of the physical form in the embryo and then maintains the adult form through its hydraulic, electrochemical, and spiritual power. Formless water assumes whatever conformation is required and transmits information according to its internal organization. It carries the dynamic power for change that spirit brings, unlike the fixed connective tissue structures whose shape is relatively determined.

In this chapter, we explore how the oscillation of potent fluid creates and maintains the shape of its solid container. The connective tissue container composed of fascia and the extracellular matrix displays charge and shape, the two defining characteristics of piezoelectricity. The potency of the fluid resupplies the requisite charge to vivify and maintain the conformation of the container. Without charge, the shape collapses. Without the container, electrostatic holographic patterns cannot be fixed in three-dimensional space.

Essentially, connective tissue is "osteopathic tissue." As we will see, it expresses the precepts of the osteopathic philosophy by demonstrating unity of function, a structure-function interrelationship, and the elements necessary for its maintenance and healing. If we treat the connective tissue, we treat osteopathically.

However, because water transfers the life force to the connective tissues, we can also consider the fluids when treating. Water, too, demonstrates all three of the osteopathic/natural principles we have mentioned: a unity of function, a structure-function interrelationship, and a healing capacity. Further consideration of these concepts comes later.

Further, to be truly holistic in our orientation as osteopathic physicians, we must address energy or spirit as it engages the material aspect through water. Unlike many osteopathic physicians today, Still considered this spiritual level of osteopathic treatment fundamental to everything that he did therapeutically.

The remainder of this chapter explores the nature of both water and connective tissue. These two elements act to bring about the union of the Celestial and Terrestrial in the creation of biogen. According to Still, Life and Matter reciprocate to form biogen. In the physical, this is demonstrated by the characteristics of water and connective tissue.

At the heart of this book is Still's central thesis that spirit is fundamental to life and therefore to his philosophy. Sutherland asserted that the primary respiratory mechanism is a manifestation of spirit. He described this palpable motion, the tide, as an expression of the Breath of Life. Thus, by palpating the primary respiratory mechanism, the osteopathic physician experiences the primary effects of spirit firsthand. The thrust of this book supports Sutherland's assertion. From here, the text elucidates the interface between spirit and matter, the mechanisms of spirit's activity that manifest in the physical.

The interface between spirit and matter in the living human exists by evidence of what we feel in the tissues, the fluctuation of the primary respiratory mechanism. What is this palpable experience in terms of the anatomy, physiology, and biochemistry of the tissues? A substantial portion of this chapter is dedicated to this topic.

Before the development of the rest of this chapter, we must review two important caveats concerning spirit versus religion and spirit versus mechanics. It is fair to restate what is stated in Chapter One, that in this book, "spirit" refers to the energetic, unseen reality without the cultural attachments and dogma of religion. Relative to mechanism, we are confronted with two worldviews: one declares that we can explain all physical phenomena by understanding physical mechanisms, while the other reminds us that all mechanisms are manifestations of the effects of spirit. Inherent in this book is the concept of vitalism (spirit), which has been largely forgotten in lieu of the deterministic scientific method (mechanics).

In some sense, science is our religion. We have come to trust that, by looking deeper into the minutiae of the mechanics of things or by looking farther away to the depths of the universe, we can expect to find the answers to fundamental questions about our existence: "Who and why are we?" Science, we believe, will explain for us the logical answers to these spiritual questions. That is, we expect that, by dissecting the material aspect, the spiritual aspect will reveal itself.

In truth, according to Still, mechanisms manifest spirit. Mechanisms are the means used by matter through which spirit imparts its urge for motion in physical life. Motion in the physical realm is evidence of the intention of spirit in the ethereal realm—reciprocity of Mind and Matter. Although it is attractive in the view of the reductionistic thinker to believe that mechanisms hold the ultimate answer, Still did not believe this. He said that blood and nerves carry the influence of spirit to all parts of the body. The fluids of the extracellular space and fascia are the dwelling places of spirit.

In Still's osteopathic philosophy, science is merely the tool to uncover the mechanisms of spirit that act in the physical realm. We describe these mechanisms through astronomy, physics, physiology, biochemistry, and the other disciplines of science.

This chapter demonstrates how the physical world accommodates and integrates the influence of spirit to move elements that we understand from our experience to be material, that is, to have substance, volume, and mass. Of course, behind the illusion that matter is substantive is quantum physics shouting that matter is merely a special case of energy. Matter is ephemeral, winking on and off, into and out of existence in the explicate order, emerging as intermittent, individual, elementary particles that are mirrored as waves in the unseen realm of the implicate order (see Chapter Two).

In William Tiller's model, matter particles exist in direct space, and matter waves exist in reciprocal space. If matter is truly condensed light—merely another representation of energy—we can appreciate that energetic effects can easily influence matter. Some of these energetic effects include thought, emotion, intention, and other less tangible influences. It is time we receive this message from quantum physics and integrate it into our worldview and into our perception of the mechanisms of healing. It is the contention of Still and of this author that all physical motion derives directly from a basic force in all of creation—the life force—which emanates from spirit.

Spirit resides in the implicate order (Bohm), the reciprocal (wave) space (Tiller), or the Celestial (Still). Matter resides in the explicate order, the direct (particulate) space, or the Terrestrial. The two elements—spirit and matter—reciprocate to create a material form. Consciousness directs the process. The question the rest of this book explores is, "How does spirit *interface* with matter?" First, we explore how spirit enters the realm of the physical through the agency of water.

III. WATER: REPRESENTATIVE OF SPIRIT

A. Water Behaves as a Unit

We are all familiar with hydraulic forces as demonstrated by machines that do work. A piston in one part of a closed system drives another piston at the far extreme of the pipe because the water (or other fluid) contained within the machine has unitary action, not allowing any compression within the liquid.

Similar to human-made machines, the "earth-suit" in which each of us resides is a closed system with respect to the resonance of water (taking into account imbibing and excreting events as the means by which the container exchanges with its environment). Just as water behaves as a unit within any pond, so, too, it behaves as a unit in an organism, a container of life.

The unitary motion of large bodies of water, such as the tides of the ocean, has a counterpart in the living organism. The fluid in human bodies moves as a unit at times, especially under the healing influence of osteopathic manipulative treatment. Cranial osteopathy engages and entrains the tide. Sutherland contended that the tide manifests the Breath of Life, his term for spirit in action within the organism.

B. Water's Structure Implies Its Function

Water molecules combine two hydrogen atoms with one oxygen atom in an arrangement that looks like Mickey Mouse ears, the two hydrogens forming the two "ear" bumps on the circular head formed by the oxygen atom (see Fig. 4.1). The angle between the hydrogen atoms is about 104°, so their positive charges dominate at that pole of the molecule. The opposite (negative) charge rules at the opposite pole of the molecule, where two unbound electrons exist on the oxygen atom. Therefore, the water molecule is a strong dipole, a double positive charge on one side and a double negative charge on the other. Because it is such a strong dipole, water has very interesting chemical characteristics.

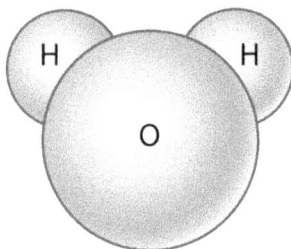

4.1   Water molecule. Original art by Raychel Ciemma.

The hydrogen atoms of a water molecule react with the oxygen atoms of two other water molecules, creating hydrogen bonds. The hydrogen bonds between water molecules are weaker than the chemical bonds between the hydrogen and oxygen atoms of the same water molecule in which electrons are shared. Nevertheless, hydrogen bonds, electrostatic in nature, impart important characteristics to a volume of water that distinguishes liquid and frozen water from other substances found in nature.

Hydrogen bonds prefer a tetrahedral pattern around a water molecule because of the tetrahedral orientation of the electrons around the oxygen atom (see Fig. 4.2). This tetrahedral pattern is rigid in the crystal structure of ice. With the increased thermodynamic energy of liquid water, the hydrogen bonds become more fluid and distorted. Water in the liquid phase does not demonstrate a rigid crystalline lattice, and the water molecules slide past each other in close proximity, enabled by distortions in hydrogen bonding. As the temperature of the water falls below 4°C, the hydrogen bonds begin to rigidify, separating the water molecules slightly into a crystalline lattice, which is set at 0°C.

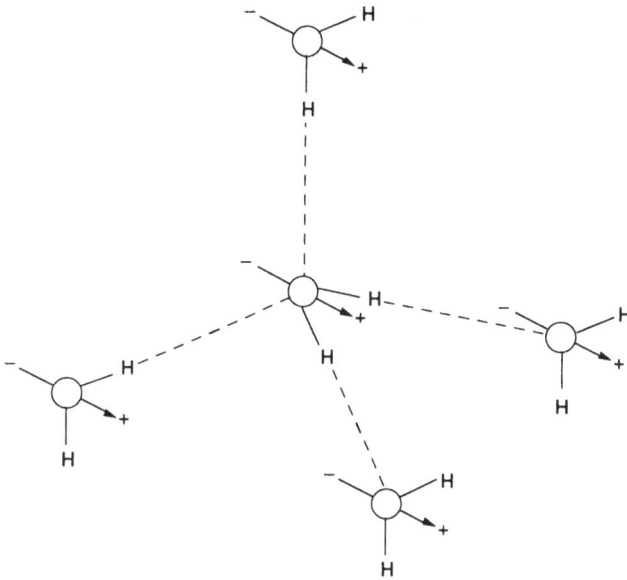

4.2   Water in ice. Five water molecules are shown in a typical tetrahedral pattern found in ice. The dotted lines represent hydrogen bonds between the separate molecules. (Reproduced with permission from Tiller WA (1997). *Science and Human Transformation*. Walnut Creek, CA: Pavior Publishing. Fig 6.5, p. 244.)

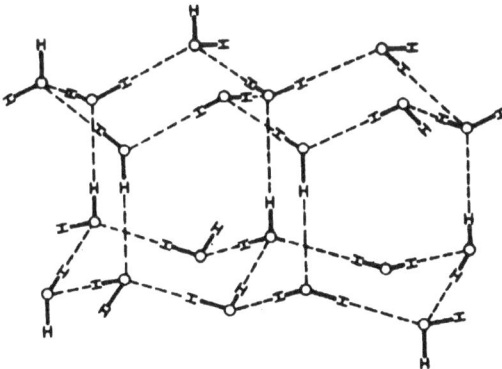

4.3   Hexagonal ice crystals. This diagram shows how water molecules relate to each other through hydrogen bonding (dotted lines) in solid ice. (Reproduced with permission from Tiller (1997). *Science and Human Transformation*. Walnut Creek, CA: Pavior Publishing. Fig. 6.6, p. 245.)

Although two or more water molecules rarely associate together in the gaseous phase, in both the liquid and solid phases of water, hydrogen bonding creates a strong affinity among molecules of water. A typical water molecule attracts two oxygen atoms from two other water molecules to its two hydrogen atoms while attracting two hydrogen atoms from two other molecules to its single oxygen atom.[2] Hydrogen bonds, even when severely distorted, as they are in a volume of liquid water, nevertheless impart important characteristics that determine water's behavior.

Molecules of water continually work to decrease the distortion of the hydrogen bonds within its matrix, favoring an orderliness of its inner structure. Hydrogen bonds create chains, brackets, and other polymers of water molecules. Although very malleable in the liquid phase, hydrogen bonds are stable enough to give a particular volume of water a character that persists as long as the physical conditions of temperature, salinity, and pH, for example, remain stable.

Molecules of water arrange themselves around ions to dissolve them. The negatively charged oxygen atoms encircle a positive ion, such as sodium, while the hydrogen atoms orient toward a negative ion, such as chloride. To integrate hydrophobic substances into water, the molecules of water form what is referred to as "structured water," in which the water molecules separate themselves from the uncharged lipophilic molecule in a bracketed arrangement, lacing together the water molecules by pentagons of hydrogen bonds.

Structured water, less dense than unstructured water, exists next to all hydrophobic membranes, inside and on the surfaces of cells, surrounding collagen fibers, and around enzymes and other physiologically active elements of the cell. In nature, structured water occurs to a greater or lesser degree according to the ionic content of the water. Potassium is especially important for the formation of open lattices of pentagons of water molecules. Spring water is often the most highly structured of all natural sources. The bond angles of structured water become visible in snowflakes and other crystallized forms of frozen water. Distilled water, on the other hand, does not form well-defined crystals. It is not structured at all.[3]

Because of hydrogen bonding, water always seeks to become spherical, creating raindrop configurations when droplets fall toward the earth. Droplets, when in contact with a surface, form quasi-hemispheres, shapes as close to a sphere as gravity and the surface allow. Capillary activity and characteristically high surface tension are explained by water's hydrogen bonding, which attempts to retain its spherical integrity, drawing its molecules together, even upward against gravity in capillary action.

Water is capable of retaining in solution most substances, hydrophilic or hydrophobic, either by dissolving them or suspending the particles, as in colloids. Water covers all surfaces on Earth, wetting them. It finds its way into the smallest places, even to be incorporated into the quaternary structure of enzymes, nucleic acids, and other macromolecules.[4]

Experiments have demonstrated that water is responsible for some physiological functions of proteins. For example, elastin depends on the nature of water for its springiness. With increased thermodynamic energy, water disengages from its intimate relationship with the tertiary structure of the polypeptide chain of elastin, allowing the helical structure to tighten its coils together. Urry actually measured elastin lifting a weight as heat was applied. This is counterintuitive because increasing thermodynamic energy is associated with increased entropy and decreased organized activity such as a tightening helical coil. In this case, however, with increased thermodynamic energy, water is driven away from its position between the helical turns where it holds apart the spirals, thus, allowing the overall length of the helical fiber to compress, shortening the overall length of the fiber to lift a weight.[5]

For these reasons, water is the most unusual substance on Earth, even though it is the most common, covering about 70 percent of

Earth's surface. It retains heat better than almost any other substance and determines weather patterns. While the sun shines, cooling winds rush to the lighter air that is more quickly warmed over land. By night, winds return to the ocean, where the air, due to the influence of the water, is now warmer and less dense.

C. Water Is Healing

1. Ice Supports Life

Water is the only naturally occurring substance that exists as a solid, liquid, and gas under conditions that support life. What's more, frozen water forms crystalline structures that are less dense than liquid water, much like the arrangement of molecules in structured water. Because of this, ice floats, a very unusual characteristic compared to other solids common on Earth. By floating, ice demonstrates how water conserves life.

If ice were heavier than liquid water, as most solids are when compared to their liquid phases, the colder surface would not protect the underlying liquid and soon it all would become a frozen solid. "All the water basins of the earth would gradually fill with ice from the bottom upwards and the earth would be transformed into a frozen waste."[6]

By expanding when frozen, water favors life in another respect. "Water that has seeped into the nooks and crannies of cliffs expands as it freezes, thus cracking the hardest rocks. In this way it starts off the dead, hard element on its way back to life." Because of this action of water, the rocks crumble to a finer and finer consistency through the course of time and become the basis for plant growth, entering into the great cycle of living nature (Schwenk, 73). And, of course, plants nourished by this soil from rock add their matter to the next layer of sedimentary rock.

The structure of water, like the structure of humans, explains its function. We can examine the surface of bones to deduce joint angles, muscle attachments, and vessel penetrations and ultimately to understand how the bone moves relative to its neighbors and what function it performs in life. So, too, we can examine the mechanical aspects of a water molecule. In doing so, its behavior in association with its neighbors emerges. Rocks break apart because, as water freezes, the hydrogen bonds that readily deform in the liquid phase become a rigid lattice created by tetrahedrally arranged hydrogen bonds, electrostatic forces with enormous mechanical consequences. Electrostatic charge is responsible for the rigid arrangement of the hydrogen bonds in solid water. Therefore, electrostatic energy moves mountains and creates soil. Energy from the ethereal realm works to support life in the physical realm.

2. Water's Flow Gives Life

Flow is inherent in water. Flow promotes exchange and is life giving. The conformation of tissues of the human body, in some cases, demonstrates the tendency for water to flow. "Both muscles and vessels speak of the same thing: streaming movement in spiraling forms. This movement runs through the sinews into the bones. The bone has raised a monument in 'stone' to the flowing movement from which it originates; indeed one might say that the liquid has 'expressed itself' in the bone" (Schwenk, 25).

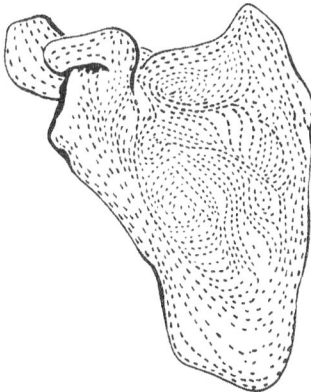

4.4   Water's flow seen in scapula. See text for explanation. (Reproduced with permission from Schwenk T (1996). *Sensitive Chaos*. 2nd. Ed. London: Rudolf Steiner Press. Figure of scapula, p. 25.)

If one makes small holes in decalcified bone and fills them with colored liquid, in time these deposits of color will lengthen out, revealing the directions of tension in the bone. An otherwise hidden system of currents in the bone are made visible outlining the conformation of the fibers of collagen (Schwenk, 25); (see Fig. 4.4).

An underlying spiraling process remains clearly recognizable in the finished forms of vessels, muscles, ligaments, sinews and bones. The same flowing movement can be detected in all these tissues, demonstrating how they are constructed (Schwenk, 26).

Fluid activity is inherent in bone. In bone's formation, collagen is laid down in fluid according to the mechanical forces inherent in embryological development, as well as in the activities of growth and healing. In the mesoderm of the embryo, at the base of the forming skull, compression occurs as the neural tube (ectoderm) expands and folds over the base from above. Simultaneously, the expansion of the developing cerebral hemispheres creates a tension in the mesoderm above the base, in the developing calvarium.

The compression below and the tension above the developing brain produce two different kinds of bone, one formed in cartilage (compression), and one in membrane (expansion). These two types of bone exhibit two different functions as a result. The motion of these two types of bone, an expression of ongoing spiritual influence, differs according to its original construction.

If, through trauma, the bones are altered from their original relationships, their function is altered as well. As osteopathic physicians, we can recreate originality to restore the inherent function by working with the intended functions of these bones, and we can use fluid to do it. After all, fluid flow delivers the necessary constituents for healing; fluid drives bony motion; and it corrects abnormal motion. We must understand the fluid nature of bone to impart health to it.

Further effects of the fluid character of bone are apparent in the fully developed organism. Bone is filled with blood, to which the profuse

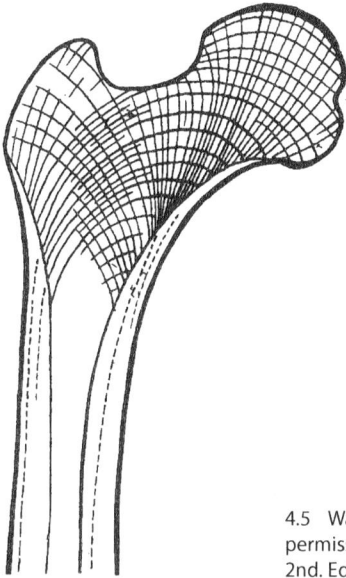

4.5   Water's flow seen in femur. (Reproduced with permission from Schwenk T (1996). *Sensitive Chaos.* 2nd. Ed. London: Rudolf Steiner Press. p. 26.)

bleeding during orthopedic surgery attests. Within the marrow of hard bone, fluid blood is formed.

The remodeling of bone is ongoing. Cowin and associates[7] identified mechanisms that remodel bone. They indicated that fluid flows and the accompanying charges within the fluid affect the stretch-sensitive receptors on the osteocytic cell membranes. Remodeling recreates in real time the evidence of normal and abnormal stress. Osteophytes are examples of bony growth into ligaments that sustain abnormally increased tension. The remodeling of osteophytes is possible with the relief of the increased strain through the application of osteopathic manipulative treatment. The orthodontist takes advantage of the fluid nature of bone to move teeth with braces.

These lines of stress follow spirals of flow, abundant examples of which exist throughout anatomical specimens in all vertebrates. The calcified deposits in the human trochanter provide a good example of spiraling flows of lines of stress within and across joints (see Fig. 4.5). The insertion of Sharpey's fibers as an extension of tension from the tendons and ligaments into the bony matrix demonstrate the continuation of flow between the outside and the inner construction of the apparently rocklike osseous scaffolding.

Dr. Robert Becker pointed out that "Stress-related bone growth is actually remodeling the shape of a bone so that it can better resist mechanical stress."[8] Under the stress of running, for example, femurs receive the jarring of repeated footfalls by minutely flexing, thus absorbing this pounding energy within the collagen and water of the system. With each deformation, collagen within the bone's structure generates an electric current. This manifestation of Still's highest known force regularly remodels bone. This is how collagen shapes the physical structure through information transmitted by water, spirit's messenger.

Another example of the activity of spirit's messenger occurs with injury to tissue. A charge is developed at the site of injury in bone or any connective tissue. The healing of injuries to tissue, such as fractures in bones, sprains in ligaments, and strains in muscles, depends on injury potentials. The injury to tissue results in catabolic activity, which is associated with a more positive potential in the surrounding interstitial space and blood plasma.[9–10]

Accordingly, the degeneration of tissue precedes and prepares for its regeneration. The controlled destruction of the injured tissue is necessary for healthy reconstruction. Without the development of an injury potential, non-union fractures result. In the healthy process, the more positive charge of catabolism is followed by the more negative charge of anabolism.[11]

The embryo, the ultimate expression of ebullient life in the physical realm, is very fluid. It floats in water, consists almost entirely of water, and initially creates the distinct forms of its tissues and organs out of water. In the beginning of tissue and organ development in the embryo, little substance is evident. Instead, differing regions of fluid take shape as precursors of the solid structures to come. The characteristics of the fluid—its salinity, its charge, and its chemical constituents—create microenvironments for the differentiation that will be expressed in the solid phase. Limb buds grow by sending out charged fluid forerunners into which cells migrate to claim new ground from the external environment for the individual taking shape.[12]

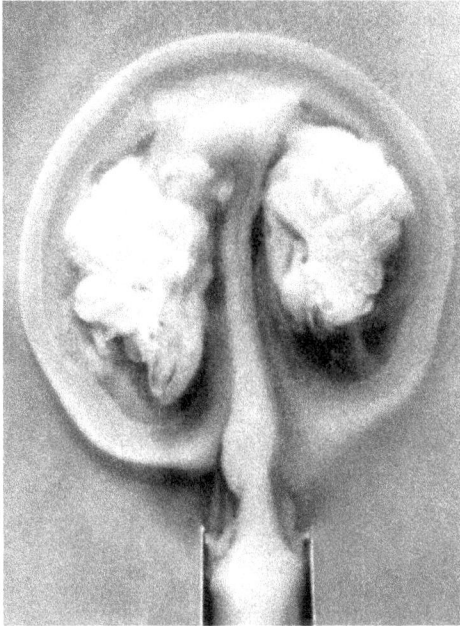

4.6   Water injected into clear, still water. (Reproduced with permission from Schwenk T (1996). *Sensitive Chaos*. 2nd. Ed. London: Rudolf Steiner Press. Plate 48.)

Schwenk photographed remarkable formations produced when colored water is injected into clear, still water. These images reveal life-like forms that result from the normal, natural flowing activity of water (Schwenk, plates 46–54). Thus, moving water demonstrates a natural urge to create embryonic forms. The corollary is also true: Embryonic forms exist because of the ordinary behavior of the flow of water[13] (see Fig. 4.6). Once again, we have evidence of spirit's impulse to create life, that is, the form of an organism.

Of course, some other physical element in addition to formless water must entrain with water's lead to develop a lasting structure. Cells migrate, compress, stretch apart, change their metabolic activity, develop intercellular communications and novel secretions, and otherwise capture the intent of the message delivered by the water from spirit's image or morphogenetic field to create an embryo that succeeds in developing a lasting form. Here we see how form follows function, with water as the intermediary.

Schwenk emphasized that the fundamental characteristics of water are consistent with the fundamental characteristics of living organisms: "all is purely functional and without fixed form" (Schwenk, 84). These qualities that both water and living systems reflect, he enumerates as metabolism, sensitivity, and rhythmicity.

3. Water's Metabolism Promotes Life

The dissolution and transmission of substances within water reveal the first function, metabolism. Salts and silt are carried or precipitated according to the conditions imposed on a particular body of water at a particular time. By dissolving solid substances, water becomes a medium of transport for nutrients and a purifier of waste. It also supports life by its characteristic of buoyancy, by which, for example, fresh silt is deposited, replenishing fruitful fields. Life is inconceivable without water. "Constantly dissolving and solidifying, washing away and re-forming, in perpetual transformation, water is everlastingly creating the organism of the earth planet" (Schwenk, 78). In the great organism of Earth and in each separate living creature, water is active in metabolic processes. Water is chemically neutral and therefore has a multitude of possibilities for nearly all chemical changes.

In the human body, water's metabolism is seen when water participates in dissolving and transporting nutrients, ions, and wastes. Anabolism and catabolism depend on water for its mediating and dissolving qualities. The breakdown of foods to usable elements through digestion depends on water's ability to dissolve. The use of these digested nutrient substances to create cells and to build up tissue depends on water's ability to distribute. It is only because water flows and dissolves solids that humans can take solid foods at all. The first, and often times the last, nourishment taken by a human consists of liquid.

Water participates not only in these transformative processes of metabolism but also in important functions of heat transfer. The amount of heat needed to raise the temperature of water by one degree is not the same over the whole range of the thermometer. It is interesting that at 37°C—normal human body temperature—water is most easily warmed. Its greatest ability to fine-tune the body's temperature is at body temperature (Schwenk, 81).

4. Water's Sensitivity Receives Life

Water's response to environmental influences demonstrates its sensitivity. It responds to influences as broad as temperature, light, chemical forces, and mechanical forces with increased or decreased viscosity, rhythms of movement, and vortices. It responds to gravity, sound, and sun with plunges off cliffs, ripples, and currents. At the surface or boundary of water, we observe its sensitivity. Differences in salt content, temperature, and alkalinity affect the merging of two bodies of water. At the surface of contact, one body rolls in on the other, creating a vortex. "A rhythmical process sets up, which evens out the differences allowing them to merge. Water is the element that brings about a state of balance everywhere" (Schwenk, 83).

"Every water basin, whether ocean, lake or pond, has its own natural period of vibration. This varies according to the shape, size and depth of the basin . . . It is like a 'note' to which the lake is 'tuned'" (Schwenk, 30). As the moon or sun influence the water basin by a pull of gravity, this pitch of the pond resonates with rhythmical vibration, creating tides and waves. The same can be said of the human body—each has its own inherent resonance. That resonance can be palpated and manipulated to assist its own urge for unity and balance.

Projections of a body of water, like bays and estuaries, behave like fingers for the sensitive detection of environmental influences—

chemical, mechanical, or thermal changes—and then transfer this information to the rest of the body of water for its integration. We see currents produced by thermoclines, salinity differences, or pressure gradients that move through a body of water, representing an activation of its sensitivity.

Water is most able to receive information from its environment when it is in motion, especially when it has been shaken. An experiment during an eclipse demonstrated the effect of sunlight on the transmission of growing potential to plants. Labels were placed on containers of water recording the extent to which each was exposed to sunlight as the eclipse progressed and receded. Each container was rhythmically shaken at the time recorded on its label. The containers of water were then used to germinate wheat seed under otherwise identical conditions. Seeds germinated in water that had been shaken when the eclipse was at its peak did not grow well. However, seeds germinated in water that had been shaken in full sunlight grew well (Schwenk, 65–66).

In homeopathy, succussion (shaking) is an important process in preparing remedies. Traditionally, the homeopathic pharmacist employs succussion in preparing homeopathic remedies, striking a container of the fluid on the palm of his or her hand one hundred times for each successive dilution. Succussion fixes the potency of the remedy, the passage of the potency from one dilution to the next, and the incremental advancement of the potency with each successive dilution.

In the body, the sensitivity of water determines the receptivity of all the sensory functions. All the sense organs depend on water's sensitivity to carry out their functions. The ear uses water in the semicircular canals and the cochlea to transmit information to the nerve endings. The nerves also use characteristics of water and dissolved elements (minerals) to carry the message farther.

Water's sensitivity also contributes to its ability to mediate between Celestial and Terrestrial, heaven and earth, implicate and explicate, energy and matter, function and structure, thought and deed.

Recall that Masaru Emoto,[14–15] a Japanese scientist, photographed microscopic frozen droplets of water after exposing them to different influences (see Chapter Two, Section V.B). He demonstrated that water takes on the character of energetic influences around it, a beautiful snowflake pattern of a droplet from a container labeled "Mother Theresa" and an ugly pattern from a container labeled "Adolph Hitler." These experiments by Emoto created effects similar to those in which seedlings sprouted better in shaken water that had been exposed to fuller sunlight. However, a profound difference between the germination experiments and Emoto's experiments revolves around the influence of mind, intention, thought, and spirit. Whereas the germination experiments can be explained on the basis of a physical influence, sunlight, Emoto's work challenges the belief that thought does not have an effect in the physical realm. In fact, Emoto demonstrated that the vibration of thought participates in the structural arrangement of water molecules.

The relationships of water molecules to each other are determined by a vibration held in the implicate order (a thought) which then reveals itself in the explicate order (in the crystalline pattern of the water). Thoughts are vibrations of energy that create impressions on physical substance. In fact, thoughts themselves are things. As Still said, Mind is a substance. David Bohm and William Tiller agreed that consciousness has mass.

William Tiller (see Chapter Two, Section II.I) introduced new concepts, based on mathematics and physics, that mind, spirit, and emotion exist in the reciprocal space or wave space in which light travels at the square of the speed of light. The particulate space or material realm operates at the speed of light (not squared) and contains what we are familiar with in our everyday reality. Tiller emphasized that the wave space is just as real and mathematically determined as the particulate space. We can calculate events in the wave space using Tiller's mathematics just as we can calculate ordinary events of material reality.

Further, influences in the wave space can affect the particulate space and *vice versa*. Mind affects matter, according to Tiller's model.

Likewise, David Bohm (see Chapter Two, Section II.H) described two realities, the implicate order and the explicate order. He used quantum theory, but he did not apply mathematics to prove it, as Tiller did. He came to his conclusions through thought experiments, as Einstein did.

The power of Emoto's findings is phenomenal. The implications of his findings impact the central thesis of this book. His research demonstrates that mind over matter is real. By extrapolation we can conclude that indeed morphogenetic fields can shape organisms, that homeopathic remedies can transfer an energetic stimulus to the living organism through the structure of water, that water indeed transfers the influence of mind to the physical realm, and that water mediates between heaven and earth. With Emoto's experiments, we have evidence for the belief that the Love of God enters the human form through the agency of water and that water is the basis of life.

The morphogenetic field, a template of the physical form of living things, is holographic. A hologram, by definition, exists in space as a three-dimensional image, which is projected by coherent light from an interference pattern that has been developed on a physical object, such as a plate of glass (Chapter Two, Section I.B.4: "Holism"). This three-dimensional image is a field or a pattern of charge that is capable of transferring its orientation to physical matter for its own arrangement. The pattern of charges creates an effect across dimensions—from the implicate to explicate order (Bohm), from wave space to particulate space (Tiller), or from the Celestial to the Terrestrial (Still)—without respect to space and time. I believe that the morphogenetic field exists in another dimension and uses water as the medium to transduce its effects into our ordinary three-dimensional reality.

As Tiller indicated, both Newtonian physics and quantum mechanics do not allow for human characteristics. There is no place in these disciplines for thought or emotion. Quantum physics acknowledges that the observer has an influence on experiments, but there is no means to calculate such effects. Tiller's model of physics includes intention, emotion, thought, and spirit in the reciprocal space. There, in the reciprocal space, we find for the first time the opportunity to measure these previously unmeasured human qualities. Furthermore, these aspects of Mind can be related to physical form.

Because of its sensitivity, water is able to transfer vibrations of thought, intention, emotion, and spirit. Such information is passed on through the arrangement of the water molecules, determined by hydrogen bonding, which is registered in the pattern of the water crystal. The thought pattern is holographic, and the pattern carried by the water likewise is holographic.

If consciousness is material, as Still, Tiller, and Bohm proposed, then, its vibration affects the arrangement of water molecules in three dimensions. The water passes on this three-dimensional conformation of vibration to other substances with which it comes in contact. Some substances are better able to receive this pattern than others. Connective tissue appears to represent the epitome of sensitive receptors of such information. We discuss connective tissue after introducing water's rhythmicity.

5. Water's Rhythmicity Is Its Life Element

"Cleanliness is next to Godliness." Turn the waters of life loose at the brain, remove all hindrances and the work will be done, and give us the eternal legacy, LONGEVITY. — A. T. STILL

Tides and waves manifest Schwenk's third principle of water in living systems, rhythmicity. Rhythms regularly develop in bodies of water as a reaction to a variety of stimuli. For water, "rhythm is simply its 'life element', and the more it can be active rhythmically the more it remains alive in its inmost nature. Where it is deprived of rhythm and can no longer flow freely . . . it begins gradually to grow weary and die. Then it loses its ability to mediate between heaven and earth" (Schwenk, 83).

Water carries the life force through movement. It mediates between Still's Celestial and Terrestrial. Water arranges and moves the material substance of the explicate order, transferring to it the life force from the implicate order. Motion manifests life. Motion in the explicate order is the agent of spirit from the implicate order. Water mediates this impulse of spirit and manifests it.

Swedenborg said that Life exists in the "juices between the fibres." Without water, the connective tissue container of life would not manifest the motion of life. The life force needs the rhythms of water to transfer to matter that which creates metabolism, biomechanics, and purposeful movement of a person, a society, and a biosphere. "In the living kingdoms of nature water is the bearer of the rhythmical processes—in the rise and fall of the sap in plants and in the pulsation of the bodily fluids in man and animal. Here too, it maintains within itself the manifold rhythms of the earth-organism and the universe, passing them on to the creatures of the earth" (Schwenk, 83).

Biological Fluid Rhythms. The primary respiratory mechanism, a manifestation of life, according to William G. Sutherland, is a rhythmical process. Sutherland used the term "Tide" to describe the inherent fluid fluctuation of the primary respiratory mechanism. There are many cellular oscillators[16–18] that depend on the rhythmicity of water, the primary respiratory mechanism being an outstanding example. (For more on cellular oscillators, see later discussion.)

Inherent motion, useful to the operator doing visceral manipulation,[19] reveals itself in organs that oscillate at a particular rate and in a specific direction. The encapsulated liver, for instance, rocks back and forth around a fulcrum established by the two triangular ligaments on the underside of the diaphragm, rendering a character of motion peculiar to that organ. The rhythmicity of the water within and out-side the cells sets up a periodic motion that is delimited by the liver capsule. The connective tissue envelope delimits the "water basin" of that particular organ, determining its inherent rhythm.

Each compartment that is defined by connective tissue can es-tablish its own unique rhythm. The compartment develops a rate, di-rection, and amplitude that characterize that organ according to its volume, the density of its contents, and the manner in which it is con-nected to its neighboring compartments.

Many novices to OMT easily palpate the liver motion, but they find the pancreas quite difficult to detect. Of course, a connective tis-sue capsule does not envelop the pancreas as it does the liver; rather, loose cellular aggregates collect around a poorly defined meshwork of threads and strands of connective tissue, as though the process of orga-nization had been turned inside out. Without a firm control over the contents of a compartment as in the liver, the connective tissue strands of the pancreas do not afford the organ a motion that can be as easily palpated.

This phenomenon of inherent motion of organs mirrors the rhyth-micity of natural basins of water. Ponds, lakes, and other bodies of water have their inherent rhythms that respond to environmental in-fluences that set them to vibrating. Tides demonstrate the rhythmicity of a body of water responding to its environment. Just as we can sit at a lake's edge and watch the waves lapping at the shore, so too we can watch, through palpation, water's rhythmicity in contained organs of the living body.

Inherent Motion of the Brain. The brain has its inherent mo-tion, one that Still referred to as a "dynamo." He said that the brain is a battery that develops charge by moving like a dynamo (see Fig. 4.7). Electroencephalograms and tests of oscillating magnetic fields[20] of the brain prove the existence of this dynamo activity postulated by Still.

He also commented that the dynamo of the brain starts with the action of the cerebellum. Radiographic evidence of brain motion by real-time magnetic resonance imaging (MRI) demonstrates that the cerebellum, brain stem, and diencephalon move in the directions that Still proposed a century before using no imaging technology other than his inherent faculties.

We know that the brain develops its ram's-horn configuration in the fetus. The recapitulation of the motion of the progressive growth and development of these tissues in the embryo defines the brain's inherent physiological motion in the adult, its natural resonance. The spinal cord, brain stem, and diencephalon cyclically descend and ascend. They move together caudally and then rostrally, toward the original leading edge of the embryonic neural tube, the *lamina terminalis*, situated in the adult at the anterior end of the third ventricle.

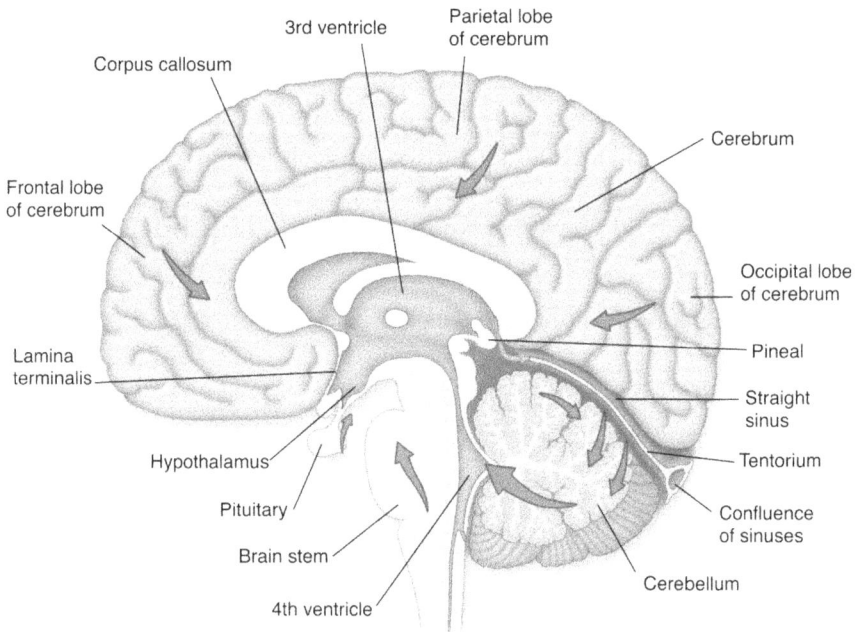

4.7   The brain as a dynamo as described by A.T. Still. Original art by Raychel Ciemma.

Cardiovascular–Central Nervous System Rhythms. Feinberg[21] reviewed the literature on brain and cerebrospinal fluid (CSF) motion in 1992 and commented that O'Connell, in 1943, had speculated that a vascular pump aids CSF dynamics, based on spinal tap measurements. In 1966, duBoulay[22] cited the third ventricle as the pump that moves the CSF. He said that brain expansion causes thalamic compression of the third ventricle with each cardiac pulse. In 1985, MRI at the Karolinska Institute in Sweden demonstrated signal intensity changes in the aqueduct as a function of the cardiac cycle.[23]

Fourier velocity imaging, developed by Feinberg and Mark at the University of California at San Francisco, demonstrated in 1986 that "with the arrival of the systolic pulse wave, internal regions of the brain moved caudad, imparting a compressive force on all three ventricles and initiating a CSF ejection." They reported that CSF is ejected caudad through the foramen of Monro, aqueduct, foramen of Magendie, and basal cisterns. CSF is ejected through the foramen magnum out of the cranial cavity and into the spinal compartment. In diastole, the flow reverses.[24–25]

With cardiac activity, Enzmann and Pelc reported in 1992 sequential motion of the brain stem and diencephalon, occurring first and with greater displacement (0.4 mm ± 0.16) in the cerebellar tonsils. They observed that both the hypothalamus and distal brain stem moved slightly later and with less displacement. Simultaneously, the brain stem and CSF quickly move just after carotid systole in a caudal direction toward the foramen magnum, followed by a less rapid recovery in the cephalic direction. The cerebral and cerebellar hemispheres move in the opposite, cephalic, direction with carotid systole.[26] Poncelet and associates also observed a compressive movement of the thalami on the third ventricle with systole.[27] Both sets of researchers observed a maximum motion of 0.5 mm associated with carotid pulsations.

These observations support Still's contention that the dynamo begins with the cerebellum. According to these radiological observations, the root of the cerebellum and its hemispheres move in opposing directions, pointing to the cerebellum as the fulcrum for this activity. It eventuates in a squeezing of the third ventricle, moving the brain stem and diencephalon caudad and the cerebrum cephalad.

Cerebrospinal Fluid–Central Nervous System Rhythms. The motion of the cerebrum has a different character than the base of the brain because of its different embryological origin. From the sides of the rostral end of the embryonic neural tube extend two protrusions (emanating through the foramina of Monro), one for each cerebral hemisphere. These hollow fingers, the developing cerebral hemispheres, grow faster than any tissue around them, including the connective tissue container to be.

Thus, these two eminences grow in an anterior direction only for a short distance, until they are forced to turn superiorly by the emerging frontal bone and dura mater. Once turned superiorly, the slower-growing container then forces them to grow posteriorly, then inferiorly, and finally anteriorly and laterally. These turns create, in order, the frontal, parietal, occipital, and temporal lobes of the cerebrum.

The ventricles, residing in the center of these developing lobes, contain CSF. The periodicity of the fluid fluctuation inside and outside the cerebral hemispheres harmonizes with the inherent motion of the cerebral tissue, which moves in cycles. The hemispheres shorten and lengthen in their long dimensions, but, twisted as they are into this ram's-horn shape, their overall motion results in the simultaneous foreshortening and widening of the cerebrum within the calvarium in one phase of motion. The reverse occurs in the other phase of motion.

Essentially, the cerebral hemispheres recapitulate their embryonic development with each cycle of shortening and lengthening of their long dimension. With each shortening of the long dimension of the curved tube of the cerebrum, the overall brain is felt to decrease its anteroposterior dimension and increase its bilateral dimension. With each lengthening of the coiled wormlike long dimension, the overall change of shape of the brain increases the anteroposterior diameter within the skull and decreases the bitemporal measurement.

Simultaneously, the brain stem, diencephalon, and cerebellum ascend with the shortening of the cerebral "worm" and descend with the extension of the long dimension of the cerebrum. Thus, we have the dynamo activity of the brain first proposed by Still. Sutherland was the first to describe this motion in detail. One and one-half centuries before them, Swedenborg first noted inherent motion in the brains of living dogs. He also recorded pulsatile ejections of the CSF from the brains of these animals at craniotomy.

These descriptions are of two different rates of motion: cardiac and primary respiration. In the living tissues, both motions simultaneously exist, making independent evaluation difficult. Motion in the brain stem has been recorded by gating radiographic equipment that has been carefully set to detect rates of motion for cardiac activity, even to the exclusion of other rates of motion. The much slower cerebral motion previously cited has been discovered by palpation and physiological studies.

Goldbeter[28] described a putative mechanism to explain how rapid rhythms and slower ones are coupled by various biochemical mechanisms. Cyclic motions of a rapid period of, say, 5 seconds can couple with cyclic motions of a slower period of 13 minutes, for example. Periodic electrical activity of the brain occurs in a range between a few milliseconds to about 10 seconds, averaging about 5 seconds. This coincides with the release of calcium by bursting activity in the brain. It is also seen in the beta cells of the pancreas. Gradually, levels of potassium build to a threshold that causes a repolarization of the system every few minutes, averaging 13 minutes in the case of the variation of the release of insulin. Thus, we see the coupling of regular rapid electrical activity with slower chemical waves.

Clinically Detected Rhythms. Using palpation, osteopathic physicians detect not only cardiac and pulmonary influences but also a slow oscillation in the tissues of the body, including the head and its contents. Radiologists looking for the best possible resolution of images have found interference from cardiac activity, but they have not looked for the slower waves, which are too slow to interfere. Physiologists looking for functional characteristics have found waves of cardiac and pulmonary rates as well as the slower ones of primary respiration.

Osteopathic physicians feel not only this primary respiratory rate of 6–14 times a minute but also a slower wave of 1–2 times a minute. James Jealous, DO, postulated that this slower palpable wave with a period lasting approximately 0.5–1 per minute represents the inherent motion of the tissue of the central nervous system (CNS), exclusive of the influences of cardiac or pulmonary activity.

Moskalenko, Frymann and associates wrote about the integration of the functions of the cerebrovascular and CSF systems.[29] In the cranial concept, both the cerebrovascular and CSF systems operate at both cardiac and primary respiratory rates. Studies by Nelson, Sergueef, and Glonek (2003) of fluid motions of the cranium detected evidence of cardiac, pulmonary, and primary respiration.[30]

What is palpated in treatment as the commonly used rate of 6–10 times per minute might be a harmonic of all of these waves of cardiac, pulmonary, and inherent influence. It might also represent a harmonic of the palpator's own rhythm with these other rhythms. Treatment might represent a resolution of the disharmonies of a multitude of various rhythms and an entrainment of them. Following a still point, we are able to detect by palpation this entrainment phenomenon in which all parts of the system oscillate in synchrony.

Metabolic Rhythms. Moskalenko and Frymann indicated that the *amplitude* of waves inherent in the cranium correlates with the volume of the fluid, whereas, the *frequency* of a particular wave relates to metabolism.[31]

Traube[32] and Hering[33] in the mid- to late nineteenth century observed fluctuations of arterial pressures in dogs at rates consistent with those reported by osteopathic clinicians. Many osteopathic physicians speculate that the Traube-Hering wave is consistent with Sutherland's primary respiratory motion. Mayer[34] repeated Traube and Hering's experiments, finding a slower wave of about 0.5–1 cycle per minute. This rate is consistent with Jealous' "slow wave," which he attributed to inherent motion of the brain.

In 1960, Lundberg studied continuous pressure recordings in the intracranial cavities of traumatized patients and found three waves, one of which has a rate that resembles the primary respiratory mechanism or the Traube-Hering wave.[35] In fact, in 1971 Jenkins et al. reported on modulations that appear to be Traube-Hering waves in the brain.[36]

Motions of the CSF that exhibit a rate of < 0.1 Hz have been recorded by investigators exploring the physiology of sleep.[37] Vern et al.[38] described continuous slow-wave oscillations (< 0.5 Hz) of cytochrome aa3 oxidation activity in the brain cortex of rabbits. These rates of oscillation resemble reports of other oscillations of cerebral blood volume and NADH redox state,[39–40] extracellular cortical pO_2,[41–45] and cerebral blood flow.[46] Vern et al. concluded from the experimental evidence that this slow oscillation of oxidative function derives from a primary metabolic phenomenon. Such oscillation, they said, signals a rhythmic regional variation in cellular oxygen consumption. They also determined that rapid eye movement (REM) sleep correlates with significant changes in oscillations of cortical blood volume and of the oxidation of cytochrome aa3.[47]

Biswal et al.[48] described a slow wave in the region of the sensory-motor cortex referable to the hand that correlated with motor activity of the hand. This motion was 60 percent greater in the gray matter than in the white matter of the cortex, implying some relationship to cellular metabolism. They noted that this slow wave is associated with changes in cerebral blood flow and blood oxygenation. In 1997, Biswal and associates reported that hypercapnia reduced these same spontaneous oscillations in the human motor cortex.[49] This implied that metabolic activity that is driven by oxidation and dampened by carbon dioxide is responsible for the motion.

Such rates of motion as those reported by Vern and Biswal correlate with those measured by Frymann[50] in 1971, in which she applied calipers and recorded the motion of the skull from cardiac and respiratory motions as well as a third motion that is slower than and independent from the first two. Later, Moskalenko and associates[51] confirmed skull bone motion with sequential x-rays and simultaneous NMR tomograms and bioimpedence measurements. They measured the active motion of the bitemporal and fronto-occipital dimensions following rapid intracarotid injection of 20 ml of radio-opaque material, and they measured spontaneous motion at the rate of from 6 to 14 cycles per minute. They calculated that the volume change under natural sinusoidal variation of pressure was 12–15 ml and that the mean amplitude of the motion was 0.38 ± 0.21 mm (maximum deviation of 1 mm).

In 2001, Moskalenko, Frymann, and colleagues reported slow oscillations of cerebral blood flow and volume ratios between the blood and the CSF within the cranial cavity. They simultaneously measured variation of blood flow, using transcranial dopplerography and blood/CSF volumes using bioimpedence.[52] The rates they observed are consistent with those that physicians palpate in the cranium when performing osteopathic manipulative treatment. In 2003, Moskalenko and Frymann reported that a manipulative technique, venous sinus drainage, altered the characteristics of the waveforms recorded in the same manner as the previous study.[53]

More recently, Nelson, Glonek, Sergueef and colleagues[54–56] reported on a series of experiments in which the measurement of the

Traube-Hering wave using an oximeter on the ear lobes of subjects coincided with observations of flexion and extension by osteopathic physicians who were simultaneously palpating the cranium of these subjects. They also reported that, following a still point, these waves become more organized. These observations support what osteopathic physicians feel in the clinic, and they support the theory that Traube-Hering waves manifest the primary respiratory mechanism.

Several verbal reports by clinicians add more evidence for the existence of a tidal movement. In rare instances when osteopathic physicians have been able to palpate the body of a dying patient, their independent observations agree that palpable evidence of tissue respiration is ongoing after the cessation of cardiac and pulmonary activity, sometimes for several tens of minutes.[57] These observations confirm the independent nature of the Tide. They indicate that the Tide is certainly primary. They also imply that the activity of the Tide could indeed represent a manifestation of the influence of spirit.

IV. CONNECTIVE TISSUE: REPRESENTATIVE OF MATTER

The fascia . . . is the "material man," and the dwelling place of his spiritual being. — A. T. STILL

A. Terrestrial Reciprocator

Connective tissue defines the living organism's container of life, the boundary, and matrix of the material aspect out of which the soul creates and continues to re-create a living individual. The connective tissue, the fundamental component of the Terrestrial, serves to receive the life force from spirit through water, thus, reciprocating with the

Celestial. The bones, fascia, basement membranes, and the extracellular matrix form the shape of the human organism, creating the space for food in the stomach, for air in the alveoli of the lungs, for blood in the sinusoids of the spleen, and for calcium in the bones.

Connective tissue creates space for the liver beneath the diaphragm and for the lungs above it. Connective tissue creates space for the brain, heart, and kidneys. The blood flows through vessels, which are shaped by and within connective tissue, and delivers nutrients to the cells that are fixed to basement membranes, elements of connective tissue. The nutrients pass through the extracellular space. This space is filled with the extracellular matrix, a living material placeholder, which is an element of connective tissue. Waste products return through this same extracellular matrix and enter the venous capillaries or the lymphatics, which are shaped by connective tissues.

Neurons, with their axonal and dendritic processes are embedded in fibrous connective tissue or in well-controlled environments of Schwann cells or nurse (glial) cells. The microglia are thought to be altered white blood cells, also elements of connective tissue.

Any motion within or of the organism involves the active participation of the connective tissue, water, and elements dissolved in water. Electrolytes that are dissolved in water drive the connective tissue to move as when muscles contract. But even tissue that does not actively contract still displays vitality through biochemical and fluid motion. (More details of this come later.)

1. Connective Tissue Segments and Unifies

I want to draw the mind of the reader to the fact that no being can be formed without material. A place in which to be developed, and all forces necessary to do the needed work. — A. T. STILL

The connective tissues—tissues of continuity—simultaneously

function to segment and to unify the organism. For example, various muscles exist as separate fascicles lying next to each other, each one surrounded by fascia to separate it from its neighbors. Yet many such fascicles are joined at their ends where the fascial compartments come together and form tendons or ligaments.

As another example, the pericardium isolates and protects the heart from its surroundings, and yet it is continuous with the cervical fascias, above, and the superior surface of the diaphragm, below, playing an intermediary mechanical role between the extremes of these fascial attachments, the cranium and pelvis. As a further example, the meninges segment various parts of the CNS and simultaneously unify its container from sacrum to cranium. Through the agency of the dura mater, the entire CNS is coordinated in contour and motion. It serves to integrate its form and function.

Humans might give a name to a particular area or layer of connective tissue to identify it as a separate entity, but it is not separate from the whole meshwork of the body's structural matrix—it is integral. Further, the fascia mediates among multiple varieties of connective tissues—including bones, ligaments, and basement membranes—in one seamless continuum.

All cells of the living organism, with the exception of the gametes and circulating blood cells, either touch, are anchored on, or are bounded by elements of connective tissue: fascia, basement membrane, or extracellular matrix. Every organ resides within an envelope of connective tissue (for example, the liver capsule) or suspends itself on a scaffolding of a fibrous network (as the pancreas does).

2. Fascia to Matrix

By emphasizing the connective tissue, modern osteopathic manipulative medicine, as opposed to medical specialties, focuses on the organism as a whole because the fascia unifies the body. We have given special names to some gross fascial structures, for example the peritoneum, the lumbodorsal fascia, and the falx cerebri. We have named histological structures such as the sarcolemma, neurolemma, and basement membrane. All of these structures are continuous with each other, unifying the organism both structurally and functionally. Recently, histologists have characterized microtubules and microfilaments inside the cells as finer representations of connective tissue, all of which function as a unitary structure.

Connective tissues unify the organism not only mechanically but also through another mechanism. Pischinger[58] indicated that a stimulus at any point is immediately transmitted through the entire network of connective tissue. A focal input has a global effect in the body by virtue of the electromechanical properties of the connective tissues. Electrostatic charge or electric currents exist in and transmit information through the extracellular matrix of the connective tissues. Mechanical effects are transmitted through the connective tissue at the speed of sound (Pischinger, 133). The extracellular matrix is one of the mediators of these effects. (See later discussion.)

3. Bone

As the most fundamental of all connective tissues, bone serves a scaffolding function in the formation and the shape of the organism. Bones are basic in the physical expression of the life force, macroscopically and microscopically. The artistry of dance and the dance of biochemistry represent two ends of the spectrum of the life force manifested in bone. The osseous structures, the hieroglyphical representation of worlds, as Still put it, form the microcosmic representation of the macrocosm, the human organism relative to the organization of the universe.

Still named his profession after this osseous substance. We can use the position and movement of a bone to diagnose and treat structural distortions related to ill health. Bone is that basic tissue responsible for the containment of the life principle, an earthly, rock-hard substance at the foundation of health. Yet, as rock-hard as it seems, bone is fluid-filled in the living body. It is constantly remodeling. Bone is pliable to a microscopic but essential degree. Looking at the remains of physical life in dried bones, we often forget this important point, that living bone is moving and flexible. When bent, bone discharges electric current; when injured, it develops an "injury potential"; and when healthy, it transmits energy through its fluid content, just like any other connective tissue.

As Swedenborg so aptly put it 300 years ago, "Life is found in the juices between the fibres." This aphorism speaks to the entire body's systems of energy, not just bone or connective tissue. But, as we will see, fluids next to or within the containers defined by connective tissue fibers are responsible for the transmission of the life force, effecting and affecting all sorts of metabolic activity. Likewise, fluids next to bilaminar membranes carry life-giving charge.[60]

Critically, bone is also the repository, as we will see, of an enormous quantity of calcium, 90 percent of the total amount of the body. Furthermore, calcium provides an essential material impetus that transfers the life force in fluids of the living organism.

B. The Vessel of Life

1. Piezoelectricity

As an electrician controls electric currents, so an Osteopath controls life currents and revives suspended forces. — A. T. STILL

The entirety of the components of connective tissue creates the form of the organism, the vessel of life. If all other tissue is extracted from the body except for the skin and connective tissue, the organism appears grossly identical to the living intact body.

Connective tissue is the out-picturing in the material realm of the effect of the morphogenetic field from the spiritual realm. Connective tissue is prepared with special characteristics to receive and express the life force. At the head of the list of these characteristics is the fact that a major component of all connective tissue—collagen—is piezoelectric.[61] Other components—various other fibers and apatite—also express this piezoelectric characteristic, although we do not discuss them here. This piezoelectric quality is simply defined as a relationship between charge and shape. When electricity is added to the system, it affects the mechanical structure. When distortion is applied to the system, it creates a current of electricity through the structure. Collagen carries a polarized charge that determines this behavior. In summary, electric current and mechanical movement are inherently related to each other in living connective tissues, and collagen, the most numerous element in the connective tissues, is largely responsible for the piezoelectric characteristic. These activities are very vibrant and changeable.

The more stationary electrostatic charge and physical shape also demonstrate piezoelectric qualities. In other words, the pattern of physical conformation contains a pattern of charge as well. This holographic pattern of charge in the connective tissues matches a purely energetic pattern of charge, a morphogenetic field. The morphogenetic field, a rather stable construction of energy like a standing wave in a river, preexists the physical out-picturing of the connective tissue. The morphogenetic field is what Still referred to as the "plans and specifications." From the hologram of the electrical field, another interpenetrating hologram—connective tissue—resonates to create the material scaffolding. The connective tissue brings into material manifestation a shape that originates in the unseen realm of energy. Collagen and the other piezoelectric elements of the connective tissues lend qualities to the fascia, extracellular matrix, and so forth that offer to spirit the possibility of existing on the material plane. Spirit uses this mechanism to build its earth suit.

From the material scaffolding (the connective tissue component of the extracellular matrix) hang the other two aspects of Pischinger's "triad of life": the parenchymal cell and the nutrient vessel. Biogen, as described by Still, satisfies the same function as Pischinger's triad of life.

Energy transfers from the spiritual realm to the physical realm and is transduced to metabolic activity as a function of electricity. Still called the electric activity of the body the "highest known order of force."

> All must have, and cannot act without the highest known order of force (electricity), which submits to the voluntary and involuntary commands of life and mind, by which worlds are driven and beings move.[62]

Connective tissue holds a charge because collagen molecules are bipolar. The arrangement of the collagen is determined by the manner in which the environment influences the molecules as they self-assemble. The collagen fibers are laid down in line with the electrical and/or mechanical forces that are present within or impinge on the tissues during development, growth, repair, and maintenance.

Thus, the positive and negative ends of the molecules organize themselves to operate efficiently in a piezoelectric—mechanical and electrical—sense. The positive ends orient themselves in the direction of growth. The flow of energy determines the mechanics of the tissues, which, in turn, determines the conformation of the collagen, which, in turn, determines the flow of energy in the connective tissue. Accompanying the conformation of collagen is a field of charge. A flow of current corresponds with collagen's mechanical ability. In health, this original structure, exhibiting fluid mechanics and the "highest known force," operates flawlessly.

In 1941, Albert Szent-Györgyi (who received the Nobel Prize in 1937 for his discovery of vitamin C) proclaimed that electronic influences moved around much more rapidly than diffusion and must be responsible for the speed and subtlety of the activities of life. He proposed that proteins are semiconductors, making proteins the regulated conductors of electricity. Szent-Györgyi was correct in predicting that proteins are semiconductors, but later it was shown that virtually all molecules forming the living extracellular matrix act as semiconductors.[63] As semiconductors, these molecules can be precisely controlled as to their ability to conduct electrons. Szent-Györgyi hypothesized that a great number of atoms could be arranged in close proximity, as in a crystal lattice, so that electrons would belong to not just one or two atoms only but the entire system. He also declared that water forms structures that transmit energy. Electricity—the flow of electrons—occurs in the network of fibers that constitute the matrix, while "proticity"[64]—the flow of protons (H^+)—occurs in the water. Thus, the system retains its equilibrium.

2. Form and Function

Life is a substance which fills all of the space of the whole universe. One of its attributes is action under all proper conditions. It gives form and motion to both physical and intellectual. — A. T. STILL

To this point, scientists have not integrated the multiple levels of information to create a single hypothesis explaining osteopathic philosophy from the point of view of the inner workings of the cell and the surrounding extracellular matrix. In this book, I am drawing on many sources of information, clinical and scientific, to create a unified theory of osteopathic philosophy.

One researcher, however, did organize multiple factors into a theory that approaches the goal of this book. Biologist and mathematician, V. D. Deshmukh (1991)[65] confirmed many propositions put forward in this book, as well as many tenets of osteopathic philosophy. He proposed a theory to explain the development of the form of organisms through dynamic fluid forces and energy patterns by taking into account all forms of energy—chemical, electromagnetic, and mechanical (sound)—acting inside and outside the organism simultaneously. Some of the well-known variables that influence these fluid patterns include internal and external temperature, salinity, proton and other ionic gradients, surface tension, hydrostatic pressures, and organic compositions. He stated that a biological process and its products form a unit of function.

Deshmukh also said that form originates from intermolecular forces. Patterns develop in the organism as a result of hydrophobic forces, hydrogen bonds, electrostatic forces, and van der Waals forces. These forces determine the internal and external fluid energy waves. According to Deshmukh, the "internal fluid energy waves are analogous to the internal waves described in oceanic waters. Waves that have their maximum energy at some depth rather than at the surface are called internal waves" (61). In the cell, such complex dynamic fluid motion is constant. "Flow of water within and surrounding an organism is the very basis of biophysical structuring and organization at many levels of complexity" (63). Further, he indicated that calcium waves and movements of counterbalancing proton flows (counterions) are examples of fluid energy flows in living systems; and he said that these flows of charged particles are related to multidimensional pattern formation. These multidimensional patterns express mechanical, electrical, and chemical work. Such work is accomplished within these networks of fields, which are anisotropic. They divide space just as cell membranes and other physical barriers do. Morphogenesis is the result of these multidimensional fields and flows.

This mathematically based postulate of Deshmukh elucidates Still's notion that underlies all osteopathic philosophy: The creation of a physical form occurs through the reciprocity of the Celestial and the Terrestrial. Fields of energy represent the Celestial, while flows represent the Terrestrial. This postulate also provides evidence that supports

Sheldrake's theory of morphogenetic fields, in which a primary force field determines the organization of the physical form. This research supports the basic notions of osteopathic philosophy that the body has unitary function and that structure and function are interrelated. It also supports Sutherland's ideas that the basis of the life of the organism is in the flow of fluids. Form is created and maintained from the flow of fluid, which concurs with Blechschmidt's embryological theories that much of the embryo's generative activities depend on forces from within and without the developing form rather than from genetics alone.

3. Celestial Reciprocator—Morphogenetic Fields

The soul of man with all the streams of pure living water seems to dwell in the fascia of his body. — A. T. STILL

Let us examine how morphogenetic fields (see Chapter Two, Section II.D: "Rupert Sheldrake") generate the shapes of living beings. Morphogenetic fields are defined here as patterns of electrostatic charge, or electric fields. Electric fields, the presence of charge in three-dimensional space, offer to the implicate order the necessary ability to create form in the explicate order through the means of piezoelectric connective tissue. The field mechanically directs the electrostatically charged molecules of the connective tissue.

Thus, connective tissue is the packaging material that generates the contour of the container for spirit's impulse to exist in a world of substance. This connective tissue container could be referred to as an "earth suit," because it allows a being to exist under circumstances that otherwise would not be possible, much as a space suit does. If connective tissue is the essence of living form and if it carries a charge, then electricity can be seen as the "highest known order of force," as Still put it. It is electricity that transfers to the explicate order the "plans and specifications" from the implicate order where the morphogenetic fields exist. Electrons flow through connective tissue, balanced by the flow of ions in the water bathing the connective tissue.

Robert Fulford, DO,[66] referred to the etheric body as the energy field within which the material body is constructed. The etheric body and the physical body interpenetrate the same space, have the same form, and directly interrelate with each other. The etheric body acts as the energetic scaffolding on which the physical body is constructed. The etheric body energizes the physical body. According to Fulford, the physical body relies on the etheric body for its health. The etheric body "channels energy from the soul, the mental and emotional levels into the physical body."[67]

The pattern of charge of the etheric body nurtures the physical body, and distortions of the one will adversely affect the other. We usually deal with distortions of the physical that become disharmonious with the etheric. These distortions of structure result in disabilities of function. We term these "somatic dysfunctions." Working with both energy and material substance is possible with osteopathic manipulative medicine, according to Fulford.[68]

The interface between the two elements of energy and matter is an effective place to evoke positive change in the organism through osteopathic manipulative treatment. Still asserted that the life force (Celestial) and the substance of the body (Terrestrial) reciprocate to form the living organism. As we will see, the extracellular matrix plays a central role in this process. "In discussions with leading anthroposophic physicians, a consensus was reached that the ground regulation system [extracellular matrix] is the morphological expression of the etheric body" (Pischinger, 78).

4. Charge and Shape in Trauma

If a force exceeding the limits of the tissues to stretch alters these healthy mechanics, forcing them out of their original arrangement, the electrical and mechanical aspects of health are also altered. Both the shape of the connective tissue container and the flow of fluid and energy are changed and usually in a manner that is not consistent with optimum functioning. As structure changes, so does function. This is somatic dysfunction.

The goal of treatment is to realign the energetic and material aspects that create the human body. Physicians frequently accomplish this by applying various forces to the material aspect such as high velocity and muscle energy techniques. We also can work with the energy to realign the physical with the original pattern by attending to the primary respiratory mechanism.

C. Extracellular Matrix

1. Basic Unit of Life

Formerly called the "ground substance" or "ground regulation system," the extracellular matrix (ECM) was also formerly considered amorphous. We now know that the structure of the matrix is quite complex. The extracellular matrix is a colloid* that favors a gelatinous state but can exist as a gel (gelatin) or sol (fluid), depending on the influences imposed on it.

Because all metabolic factors pass through the matrix to and from the cell, the condition of the matrix has everything to do with cellular function. The ECM is the "staging ground" for the cell. The health of

---

* According to *Webster's Third International Dictionary*, a colloid is a substance, such as gelatin, albumin, or starch, that, when apparently dissolved in water or other liquid, diffuses not at all or very slowly through a membrane and shows other special properties, such as lack of pronounced effect on the freezing point or vapor pressure of the liquid. A colloid is also any substance, such as an aggregate of atoms or molecules, whether a gas, liquid, or solid, in a fine state of subdivision with particles too small to be visible in an ordinary optical microscope, that is dispersed in a continuous gaseous, liquid, or solid medium and does not settle or settles very slowly, (such as the liquid droplets in a fog, solid particles in smoke, bubbles in foam, and gold particles in ruby glass.)

the parenchymal cells depends on the health of the ECM. Any change of state in the colloid occurs with a change of pH, mechanical (fluid) pressure, electrolyte and oxygen concentrations, temperature, concentration and type of toxins, and electric potential (see later discussion for more details).

Virchow claimed that the basic unit of life is the cell. Pischinger added, in addition to the cell, two other components: the nutrient capillary and the ECM. From Still's perspective, we can further add to this triad the lymph channel and the nerve ending. Today, we know that the nerves, vessels, and lymphatics all terminate in the matrix. Thus, the matrix mediates all these influences on the cell. The ECM is where the action is.

Pischinger studied the ECM in detail and gave us a perspective on it that enhances osteopathic concepts. "Sea water," he said, "is the primary regulation system of the single cell; the ion composition of the structured extracellular space of multicellular organisms corresponds to this" (Pischinger, 14). The ECM also provides a supporting and filling function; and it promotes the maintenance and regeneration of parenchymal cells. The ECM, as a unitary structure, has direct contact with all parts of the body (Pischinger, 15).

Pischinger sounded like A. T. Still when he said, "The functional connection between the capillary bed and the cell via the extracellular matrix, and its disturbances [is] the starting-point of many diseases" (16–17). In this sense, "All disease processes are of the same type" (17). In other words, the ECM participates in all types of disease processes and plays a primary function in the processes of healing as well.

2. Open System: Information Transfer

Biological systems are open and dissipative, exchanging energy with their environment. The most suitable energy form through which open biological systems create and maintain structure and organization is information input and processing. Such information is in the form of electrostatic charge and electric current (Pischinger, 19). These charges and currents exist in water and fibers of the connective tissues (Becker, 64). They transmit information in the form of molecules, ions, protons, and electrons as well as via hydrophobic forces, hydrogen bonds, electrostatic forces, and van der Waals forces.

A practical example of information input affecting structure is seen on a biochemical level as information in the form of nutrition. In food, just as in the sequence of nucleotide bases in DNA, the sequence of sugars and amino acids and the conformation of the nutrient molecules trigger metabolic activity. Glucose triggers a cascade of cell functions. Certain foods turn on specific genes that stimulate inflammatory mediators. Other foods produce effects that reduce inflammation. Omega-three fatty acids increase the type of prostaglandins that reduce inflammation. The medical literature is filled with research that points to the role of inflammatory mediators in the development of obesity, diabetes, cancer, cardiovascular disease, and Alzheimer's disease. Diets containing high glycemic indices produce more insulin. Insulin creates increased levels of inflammatory mediators. The brain responds as soon as the immune system in the gut responds to these information inputs. The entire organism is simultaneously affected.

Coherent information, no matter what form it takes, stimulates the organism. The major significance of information as a nonchaotic energy form is that it is not tied to any particular energy carrier. For instance, several forms of energy transmit sound waves for our perception. Sound waves in the air transfer mechanical information to the tympanic membrane and the auditory ossicles in the middle ear. Fluid transmits mechanical energy to the sensory cells in the cochlea, which transduces it to electrical energy via the eighth cranial nerve and, finally, to the appropriate cortical areas in the brain. Loud, sudden noises also stimulate immediate motor nerve, muscular, and adrenal excitation. Likewise, ongoing regulatory information controlling vegetative functions influences all systems, having far-reaching effects from setting muscle tone to turning on certain genes for their expression.

The ECM offers the organism the capability of information transfer. Ions move through the water in the extracellular space. Electrons move over the fibrous portions of the ECM. The ECM supports the aim of the organism to keep itself whole. Instantaneous and uniform signals are carried everywhere in the organism by connective tissue that reaches every cell (Pischinger, 19). Whatever information enters the system, its effects are uniformly felt throughout the matrix through the agency of water. Let's examine how this specialized tissue accomplishes the task of information transfer by first looking at the histology of the matrix.

3. Histology of the Extracellular Matrix

The standard view is that the connective tissues are composed of fibers, interfiber fluids, and cells of the connective tissues. Later, other elements were included by some: blood-forming organs, vessels, and capillaries (Pischinger, 17). Because the connective tissue holds and nurtures the parenchymal cell, we can also consider the parenchymal cell as an aspect of the connective tissue, an aspect in which the parenchymal cell serves as the central focus of activity. The parenchymal cell's actions and reactions are closely tied to the autonomous activity and reactive ability of the connective tissue (Pischinger, 17). The matrix of the extracellular space, or the "biological terrain," determines the milieu—pH, electrostatic charge, ion content, and delivery of nutrients and return of waste products—for the parenchymal cells. Still was describing the same cell-connective tissue relationships when he discussed biogen. Nordenström described additional functional detail of this same set of basic elements of living tissues (see later discussion for more on Nordenström).

The most abundant protein in the ECM, and indeed in the vertebrate body, is collagen. Collagen is mechanically the strongest protein, but is also somewhat adaptable to physiological changes. Hormones and physical exercise alter the construction of the collagen fibrillar network.[69] In addition to creating collagen, the fibroblasts in the ECM also extrude a meshwork of sugar-protein polymers, the majority of which are proteoglycans, followed by structural glycoproteins: collagen, elastin, fibronectin, laminin, and others.

"Proteoglycans (PGs), glycosaminoglycans (GAGs), and structural glycoproteins [collagen] form a molecular sieve through which the entire metabolism of the capillaries to the cell and *vice versa* penetrate" (Pischinger, 19). Molecules over a certain size or charge are subject to exclusion. The "pore size" depends on the concentration of the existing PGs and GAGs, their molecular weight, the types and quantities of electrolytes present, and the resultant pH.

The GAGs contain sulfated moieties that bind to a protein backbone, which in turn binds via link proteins to a hyaluronic acid backbone, forming PGs. GAGs—chondroitin, dermatan, keratan, and heparin—are heavily sulfated and consequently negatively charged. As a result, they stand out straight against the negative charge of their neighboring GAGs forming an arrangement like the "bristles of a brush." This creates a strong field or "domain" of negative charge[70] (see Fig. 4.8). Water moves into this well-organized domain and binds to the GAGs. PGs are the largest macromolecules found in biological systems. They form a gel and set up a barrier to the movement of water, ions, and proteins.

Hyaluronic acid (hyaluronan) is the most phylogenetically ancient biopolymer of multicellular life forms, and it is the first extracellular component to appear in the embryo. Hyaluronan is an extraordinarily long polymer and assumes a zigzag shape that occupies such a large volume that it overlaps other hyaluronic acid fibers. By itself, even without the binding of other GAGs, hyaluronan forms a negatively charged domain and establishes a barrier function. It is ubiquitous in the extracellular space of the organism. Hyaluronan also regulates cell division and cell movement (Pischinger, 46).

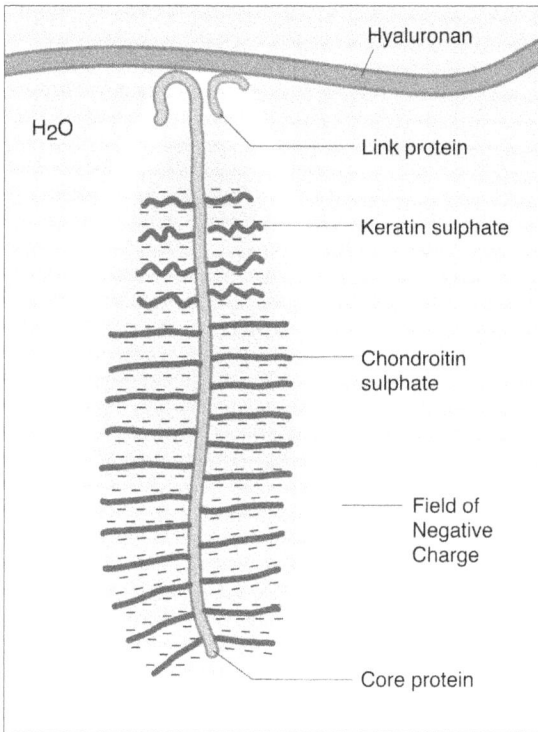

4.8 Proteoglycan molecule. Original art by Raychel Ciemma.

This negatively charged domain of the ECM operates as a liquid crystal. Networks of water molecules, through hydrogen bonding and the gel-like character of the PGs, provide the extracellular matrix with the capabilities of a semiconductor. The liquid crystal establishes a basic electrostatic tone that inherently develops parallel waves of ions that are unstable, constantly forming and dissolving and moving through the matrix (Pischinger, 52). Any variation of the electrostatic tone—ion concentration—informs the glycocalyx covering the cell membrane. This causes either the depolarization of the cell membrane, as in the case of muscle or nerve cells, or the activation of secondary messengers, such as cyclic adenosine monophosphate (cAMP), inositol triphosphate (ITP), or calcium ion (Ca^{2+}). These, in turn, stimulate intracellular mechanisms through the activation of cytoplasmic enzymes and nuclear genetic material.

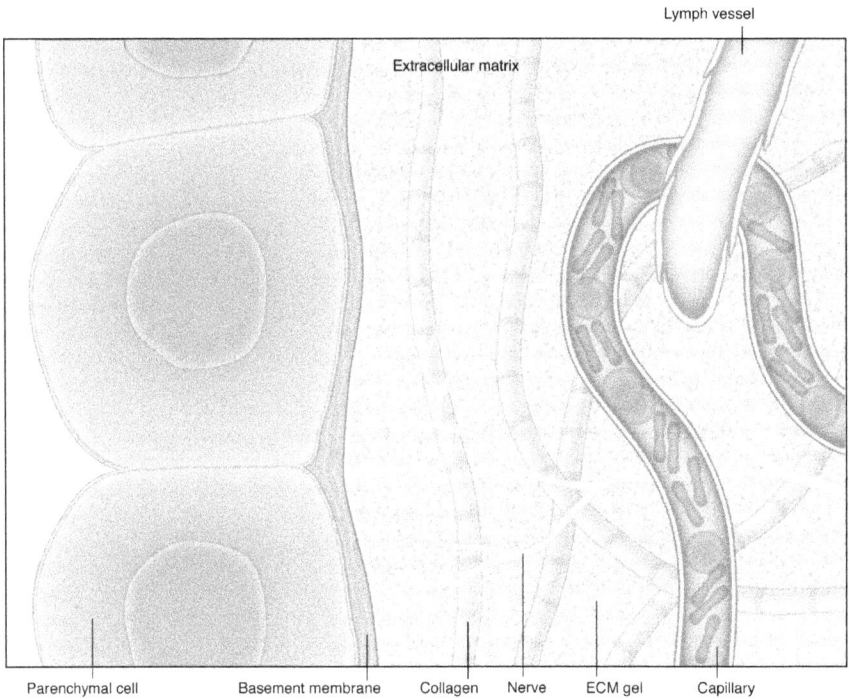

4.9   The extracellular matrix in steady state. Original art by Raychel Ciemma.

Of all the divalent cations, Ca^{2+} appears to be the most predictable in eliciting a perpendicular swelling of hyaluronan.[71] In fact, the concentration of Ca^{2+} is inversely related to the dimensions of hyaluronan polymers.[72] This has implications for the "pore size" of the matrix, allowing water and substances to flow through the matrix with greater ease as the calcium concentration and pore size increases.

Collagen Gel Contraction. A phenomenon called collagen gel contraction occurs in the ECM during conditions of inflammation and wound healing. Collagen gel contraction seems to be initiated by fibroblasts that migrate through the collagen lattice rearranging the loose-knit fibers into bundles, creating a visible decrease in the volume

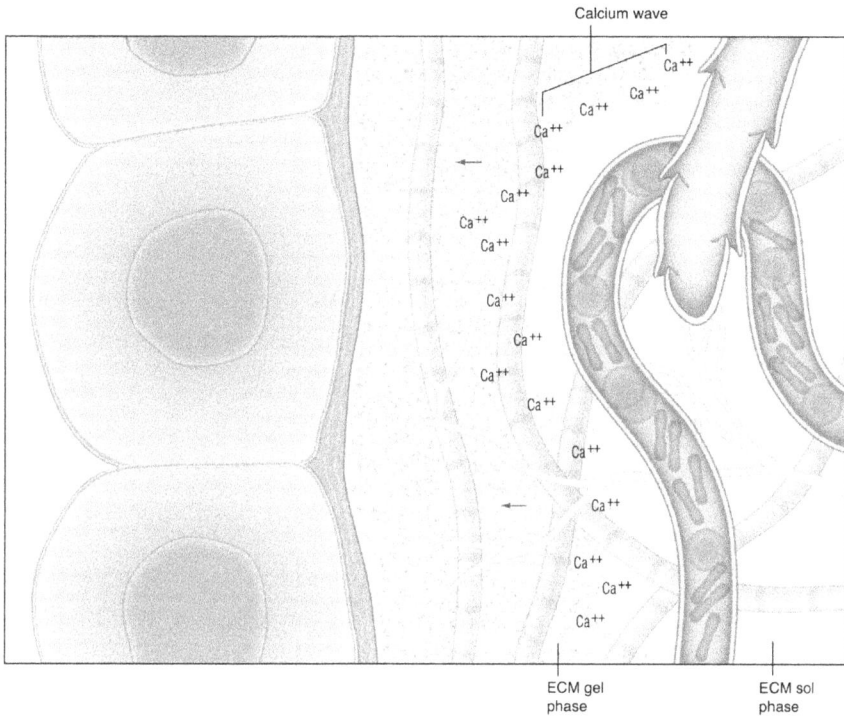

4.10 The extracellular matrix showing the influence of calcium ion waves on the depolymerization of the proteoglycan molecules. Original art by Raychel Ciemma.

of the collagen lattice. Integrins, which mediate intracellular and extracellular mechanics, have been assigned a putative role in this physiological function. (Integrins are molecules that lie within the cellular membrane and bind GAGs in the ECM as well as elements of the cytoskeleton in the cytosol. They perform essential communication functions via electrical, ionic, and mechanical means between the outside and inside of the cells; see Section IV.E: "Matrix and Cell—The Role of Integrins.) Various mediators of inflammation, including cytokines, angiotensin II, and platelet-derived growth factor (PDGF), stimulate collagen gel contraction by inducing a change in the expression or activity of integrins.[73]

Supposition holds that this phenomenon is related to palpatory changes in the consistency of soft tissues that have been chronically inflamed or that are healing. Osteopathic physicians note nodules, ropiness, trigger points, and other palpatory changes in the tissues that might represent this phenomenon in the ECM.

Homeodynamics. The ECM is related to the endocrine system through the capillaries and to the CNS through the autonomic nerves. Both capillaries and autonomic nerves terminate and function in the ECM. The endocrine and the nervous systems are connected to each other in the brain stem and diencephalon, assuring that higher centers influence and are influenced by the matrix. Further, the circulating white blood cells that wander through the connective tissues are just as "informed" as the endocrine and nervous systems. Thus, we can say that the matrix is the meeting ground for psychological, neurological, immunological, and endocrinological influences.

The matrix is a vast, complex, intermeshed humoral network. It regulates homeostasis. A better word to describe this complex activity is "homeodynamics." Homeostasis is derived from the root words *homeo*, meaning the "same," and *stasis*, meaning, among other things "a slowing of fluid flows." As this chapter describes, there is dynamic fluid activity at the cellular level on which life depends. This fluid dynamism, from the osteopathic perspective, is felt as the inherent rhythms in the tissues. Much diverse activity occurs in the ECM.

Under the control of integrins, the ECM plays a role in fluid dynamics. Integrins seem to be responsible for the state of the tension of the collagen within the ECM. Loose connective tissue naturally attracts water due to its content of hyaluronan and other GAGs. If the tension among collagen fibers increases, interstitial fluid pressure increases and water moves out of the area of compaction. An increased concentration of PDGF strongly stimulates collagen gel contraction and an increase in interstitial fluid pressure, whereas an increased level of intracellular cAMP is associated with a decrease in collagen gel contraction and a decrease of interstitial fluid pressure.

These findings demonstrate how the ECM modifies the capillary filtration rate to produce or reduce edema. The active control is likely mediated via collagen-binding β_1 integrins. This opens up the possibility that a wide range of physiological and inflammatory mediators can influence the tension on fiber networks via modulating the activity of β_1 integrin function, which in turn influences, for example, transcapillary transport and fluid balance of the loose connective tissue (Rubin et al., 288).

The energy flow in the matrix depends on the swarms of liquid-crystalline water that react with the biopolymers. The degree of organization of the matrix relies on these flows of water and its fluctuating redox potential. These fluctuations of potential describe a transformation between energy and mass and determine the conditions of energy flow in the ECM. Sutherland asserted that an energy-matter transformation happens during a still point of the primary respiratory mechanism. He taught that at a still point a transformation occurs everywhere simultaneously. His hypothesis is consistent with characteristics of the ECM, because it transmits information instantaneously throughout and it participates in transformations between energy and matter.

As palpable fluctuations in the tissues reach stillness, changes occur in the extracellular space where the "finer nerves dwell with the lymphatics than even with the eye . . . and all drink from the waters of the brain" (Still 1892, 66). The redox potential is reset everywhere simultaneously. All fluid compartments of the organism, all extracellular spaces undergo a transformation, a resetting of electrical potential. Free electrons recharge the fluids, raising the pH, which recollects vital minerals, such as magnesium, which catalyzes the production of ATP in the respiratory chain of the mitochondria.

We can hypothesize that it is just this set of parameters—electrons that stagnate or flow; water that is bound or unbound; piezoelectric polymers that polymerize or depolymerize; and counterions such as hydrogen ions, calcium ions, and other electrolytes that stagnate or flow—that determine the transformational capacity of the tissues that Sutherland discovered from clinical observation and described in 1939. Sutherland showed us how we can clinically create this transformation by inducing a still point. This resetting of the viscosity and electrostatic charge of the ECM is accompanied by a resetting of vast neurological and humoral networks of function. This allows Health to return to the tissues.

The homeodynamics of the extracellular milieu is managed by the rapid transmission and distribution of information, as opposed to the function of storage of information, which is a primary function of another important biopolymer, DNA. However, both DNA and matrix biopolymers perform both functions of storage and transmission of information.

Homeodynamics also involves the quenching of free radicals that result from normal metabolic activity. The water and sugar polymers act as a redox system, taking up and giving off excess electrons and protons in the form of oxygen and hydroxyl radicals. In the course of ATP production along the mitochondrial respiratory chain, the matrix "cools the organism's reactor," thus heating the matrix and providing energy for other metabolic reactions.

If the ground substance is not freely washed by adequate lymphatic and capillary circulation, an accumulation of free radicals occurs. Thus, we have a modern biochemical explanation for Still's declaration that poisons in the tissues are at the foundation of disease processes. Pischinger asserted that a chronic, nonphysiological alteration of the redox potential of the matrix leads to the development of chronic inflammation and the danger of the development of tumors and cancers (Pischinger, 27). Thus, we can more fully appreciate Still's pronouncement that pollution in and the fermentation of the tissues are responsible for the beginnings of disease and his consequent admonition to his students that they must treat the nerves, open the arteries, and flush the waters of the lymphatics.

4. Toxins

The matrix normally stores four types of nutrients: sugars in the GAGs and PGs, proteins as amine groups (—NH) in the PGs and collagen in the matrix, fatty acids in the membranes of the cells, and the ubiquitous water. In pathological conditions in which protein and amyloid storage is increased, many other types of substances accompany them: immunoglobulins, lipoproteins, fibrinogen-complement, albumin, environmental toxins, and antigens. The detoxification function of the liver reduces the load of the proteinaceous substances by excreting them into the bile. But when metabolic processes are high, the connective tissue—especially the matrix—receives these substances and holds them for later processing by the liver when the organism is at rest. So, the matrix can also act as a waste dump. In such cases, in which excess toxins are stored in the connective tissues, the pH is reduced, thus altering the content and activity of the alkaline minerals, especially magnesium and potassium, the majority of which are intracellular.

Further, if the autonomic nervous system is the mediator of disease, as Irvin M. Korr, PhD, so eloquently has shown,[74-75] the mechanism of that mediation is predominantly through the sympathetic nerves, ending in and consequently congesting the ECM. The secretion of norepinephrine by the sympathetic nerve endings in the ECM changes the "setting" of the viscosity of the GAGs. The biopolymers become more organized, establishing a more distinct negative electrostatic domain to which water is attracted and bound.

The rigidity of the system reaches a maximum when the GAGs have become well organized, firmly bound to the hyaluronan backbone, and fully impregnated with bound water, establishing a gel. Nutrients and waste products from metabolic activity cannot easily move through this negatively charged field and gelatinous mechanical barrier. The extracellular space develops a higher than normal concentration of waste products. The pH becomes more acidic. Calcium and magnesium ions move out of the cells into the area of lower pH in the extracellular space, buffering the acidic metabolic by-products and other toxins. Water accompanies these ionic displacements, diluting the concentration of acidic toxins and creating edema.

Because magnesium is required as a coenzyme for many of the enzymes of glucose metabolism and the production of ATP, the machinery of the cell is hampered. Fatigue is a common clinical sign. Magnesium is not the only important electrolyte affected. The movement of calcium out of bone to neutralize an acid pH in a condition of toxicity is an important cause of osteoporosis.

Because of the fluid-crystalline nature of the matrix, networks of water molecules store and transfer information between cells. Water forms liquid-crystalline intercellular bridges and carries biophoton emissions as signals. The ECM, an open-energy system, absorbs free-radical energy from metabolic processes, leading to fluctuations of energy that spread rapidly throughout the matrix because of the change in state of the liquid-crystalline water. The cell uses this change in the state of the water as information. These fluctuations are measurable as biophysical oscillations of the redox potential of the matrix.

Changes in water depend on substances dissolved in it. "Structure breakers" disturb the organization of the water polymers; these include hydrophilic compounds such as sugar, urea, and silicic acid (from silica). "Structure makers" are hydrophobic elements and gases—O_2, N_2, and CO_2—dissolved in water; such structure makers impart information to the water.

5. Information and Embryology

Embryological growth and development and the repair and maintenance of mature tissue depend on the ability of the matrix to transfer information. Jaffe[76] reviewed the fundamental role of calcium ions (Ca^{2+}) as the information input to the system, both as a means for the formation of and for the information transfer through the ECM.

The patterns of Ca^{2+} concentration determine the early development of embryos from many species that have been studied: sunflowers, protozoa, *Drosophila*, humans, and others. In light-sensitive plant zygotes, calcium concentrates at the pole opposite the direction of incoming light. Development in the zygote proceeds at an increased pace at the pole of increased calcium concentration. Actin filaments and microtubules localize in these calcium-rich zones to establish the beginnings of a more permanent, material body in the form of the ECM.

In other studies, increased levels of extracellular cAMP were found in areas of greater growth. Extracellular cAMP also raises the concentration of calcium in the intracellular fluid. Electric force is a third stimulus for the accumulation of Ca^{2+}, the concentration of potassium at the plasma membrane being a primary factor. Stretch is a fourth stimulus to the localized aggregation of Ca^{2+} and the growth of the zygote (Jaffe, 663).

The healing of severed nerves starts with the extension of neurites, pseudopods that grow into the neurolemma to reestablish axons. Microtubules assemble into water-filled extensions of the existing nerve cell. Microfilaments pull at their ends to compress them. Elongation is also established by shifting compressive loads off the microtubules and onto the cell's attachments to the ECM.[77] Limb buds extend their lengths in the embryo by exchanging the substance of the watery tip with ECM constituents.[78]

6. Information and Manufacture of Matrix

Clinical observation and research studies suggest that joint loading and motion can stimulate wide-ranging metabolic responses in cartilage, the densest type of extracellular matrix. "Immobilization or reduced loading can cause a decrease in proteoglycan synthesis and content. In contrast, dynamic loading or remobilization of the joint can increase proteoglycan synthesis and content. More severe static or impact loading often causes cartilage deterioration and can lead to osteoarthritic changes."[79]

Static compression of the cartilage leads to smaller pore size and the congestion of the tissue with a resultant flow of counterions such as H^+ and Na^+, reducing the pH of the matrix. However, the oscillatory compression of cartilage at frequencies of 0.01–1 Hz leads to the increased synthesis of PGs (Grodinsky et al., 314–315). These oscillatory rates are consistent with the healing that is associated with the described rate of the tide of the primary respiratory mechanism. Dynamic compression can induce a variety of physical phenomena, including hydrostatic pressure gradients, fluid flows, streaming potentials, and currents within tissues, especially at lower frequencies (e.g., 0.001–0.01 Hz) (Grodinsky et al., 316).

In other studies, mechanical loading of the ECM changes the production of proteases by the fibroblasts in the ECM. Proteases degrade the fibrillar components of the ECM. We also know that fibroblasts produce the components of the ECM according to mechanical loading. Thus, remodeling of the matrix is an ongoing phenomenon controlled by the effects of mechanical loading of the ECM on the fibroblasts and by the fibroblasts on the ECM.[80]

6. Gel versus Sol

Multiple influences determine not only the electrostatic charge, but also the viscosity status of the matrix. Changes in the conformation of the matrix or the flow of its components routinely occur as energy-consuming activities, usually as a part of the information-encoding function of the matrix. One form of information comes through the mechanical stimulation of the GAGs. With severe or repeated mechanical demands, the shock-absorbing quality of the GAGs changes from its lubricating sol characteristic to a firm and impenetrable gel. Overuse syndromes, in which the tissues become less pliable and painful, are examples of this phenomenon. Because autonomic nerve endings deliver regulatory substances that affect the sol-to-gel transition, we see in situations of increased psychological stress increased sympathetic nerve activity that adds to the tendency for the ECM to be a gel. Moreover, epinephrine, cortisol, insulin, thyroid hormones, and sex hormones all influence the viscosity of the matrix. And concentrations of electrolytes and hydrogen ions play an important role in pushing the balance toward the gel character of the matrix.

The relationship of the viscosity to the charge of the ECM is an example of its piezoelectric quality. In health, the viscosity and charge allow for transmission of substances of metabolism. But, as stressors enter the system, the gel state predominates, congesting the tissues. The influences that affect the viscosity of the matrix oscillate regularly, as part of the routine activities of the living process. The gel phase and the sol phase of the matrix reciprocate with each other, creating a balance of activity, a characteristic of the tissues that supports osteopathic theory and practice.

Gerald H. Pollack, in his book, *Cells, Gels and the Engines of Life,*[81] described the gel-to-sol and sol-to-gel phase transition as a characteristic of cells that cuts across many types of cell functions as an essential requirement for those varied jobs: secretion, cell migration, cell division, and muscle contraction. He indicated that the phase transition happens in an instant when there is a shift in one of the various factors controlling the internal milieu: pH, temperature, ion content, biophoton output, electrical field, and mechanical stress. A phase transition is involved in several types of responses from cells including permeability, electrochemical signals, mechanical hardening or softening, and change in shape and volume. With this information, we have set the stage for the exploration of the vital respiratory fluctuations we feel in the tissues.

D. Oscillation–Extracellular Matrix and Cells

Because open-energy systems exchange energy freely with their environments, they are unstable and prone to oscillation. In the 1960s,

Fröhlich[82–83] predicted that, on the basis of quantum mechanics, biological systems must produce coherent oscillations. As already discussed, Pischinger recognized that, in addition to the function of cellular oscillators, the matrix contains its own inherent tendency to oscillate. He indicated that the contents of the extracellular matrix (GAGs, PGs, hyaluronan, electrolytes, water, etc.) establishes within the matrix the tendency to oscillate with the right information input. Such oscillation can be measured by sinusoidal variation of many parameters, including pH, ion concentration, viscosity, hydrostatic pressure, and electrostatic charge.

As Oschman reported, "We now know that all parts of the living matrix set up vibrations that move about within the organism, and that are radiated into the environment. These vibrations or oscillations occur at many different frequencies, including visible and near visible light frequencies. These are not subtle phenomena; they are large, or even gigantic, in scale. Moreover, their effects are not trivial, because living matter is highly organized and exceedingly sensitive to the information conveyed by coherent signals" (62).

Pischinger also concluded, "The most important intracellular pacer is the rhythmic synthesis of ATP by the cell mitochondria" (43). The first to discover glycolytic oscillations were Duysens and Amesz in 1957, when they noticed oscillations in the concentration of glycolytic intermediates in yeast. They also observed that the pH oscillated. Because of feed-forward stimulation by its reaction product, ADP, phosphofructokinase drives the respiratory chain of enzymes in cycles of activity, about once every five minutes, as the ratio ATP/ADP varies.[84] The ratio of ATP to ADP is an important cellular signal that regulates the functions of energy production. This sets up the cyclic availability of ATP, which affects all other systems of enzymes and operations within the cell. However, these frequencies are in the range of minutes, whereas the palpable oscillations felt by osteopathic physicians in the clinic are in the range of a few seconds to a minute or two.[85]

Oscillations consistent with the rate of the tide of the primary re-spiratory mechanism exist within the cellular membrane, among other locations. Important oscillators in cell membranes are the cyclical production of secondary messengers, cyclic adenosine monophosphate (cAMP) and cyclic guanosine monophosphate (cGMP), and flows of calcium ions (Ca^{2+}). These secondary messengers interact with each other in various feedback loops, as well as with the production of ATP itself.[86] For example, blocking cAMP transients decreases the intrinsic frequency of spontaneous Ca^{2+} spikes, whereas inducing cAMP increases Ca^{2+} spike frequency. Transients of cAMP are absent when Ca^{2+} spikes are blocked and are generated only when Ca^{2+} spikes mimic endogenous kinetics.[87] Further, oscillations in the extracellular space depend on waves of calcium ions, the associated water, and their combined effect on the biopolymers (Pischinger, 43).

The following scenario is central to an explication of the motion in the tissues that is palpated by osteopathic physicians. Waves of calcium ions move through the tissues changing the concentration of calcium in a sinusoidal fashion. As the concentration of calcium increases, PGs and GAGs depolymerize. The quantity of free, unbound water increases and penetrates the ECM. Under this dilutional effect, the calcium ion concentration declines, causing a repolymerization of the matrix and an increase in the binding of water to the biopolymers. More details of this mechanism are discussed next. For now, let me state that it is my belief that what we feel in the tissues as the Tide is related to the waves of calcium ions and the accompanying water, which is associated with alterations in the viscosity and charge of the matrix.[88]

1. Traube-Hering Waves

In the 1860s, Traube and Hering independently measured oscillations of pressure in cannulated dog arteries at a rate of about 6–10 times per minute. This rate is consistent with that which practitioners of osteopathy in the cranial field (OCF) frequently engage. In the late 1800s, Mayer found a slower wave using the same technique. This wave, at a rate of about 1–2 times per minute, is referred to as the "slow wave" by OCF practitioners and seems to relate to the inherent motion of the CNS, according to theories of James Jealous, DO.[89] Palpation of the tissues of humans reveals oscillations at rates of 6–10 times per minute (~0.1 Hz), 1–2 times per minute (~0.5 Hz), and other rates. Sutherland called the oscillation of the cranium and other tissues the primary respiratory mechanism. Sergueef and colleagues demonstrated that cranial manipulation favorably affects the Traube-Hering wave.[90] Many authors have proposed that the Traube-Hering wave and the primary respiratory mechanism are the same.[91–95]

Guyton and Harris[96] extensively studied this phenomenon in humans and proposed that the oscillation is the result of the autonomic nervous system searching about a mean to control blood pressure. Indeed, this explanation may fit with the hypothesis of this book. As described in the previous sections, the sympathetic nerve endings in the ECM of the vasculature may be producing norepinephrine in an oscillatory manner, setting up an oscillatory behavior of the tone of the vessels via the viscosity of the ECM. Alternatively, the muscle tone of the vessels may contribute to the oscillating diameter of the vessel. A third explanation may involve the oscillatory change in volume of the extracellular space through which the vessel transits, thus changing the diameter of the vessel. All of these scenarios may be true, each being controlled by sympathetic nerves. Other possible explanations, which do not involve the sympathetics at all, may be discovered to be true through future research. For example, oscillations of electrolytes or pH may play fundamental roles. The likely reality is that all of these factors participate together, locked in reciprocating loops of influence, to operate a machinery of health-delivery to the tissues from spirit.

2. Björn Nordenström and Circuits

Nordenström [97] beautifully demonstrated that circuits of electricity flow through the blood of capillaries and the fluids of the interstitium as a means of balancing metabolic functions. He called these "biologically closed electrical circuits." These circuits may transport large quantities of ions over a long period, even though the electric gradients are minimal.

He found that oxidation-reduction reactions occur adjacent to fibrous membranes. These include the organ capsules, fasciae, dura, basement membranes, tissue septa, and cellular membranes. These tissue interfaces are a barrier to the transverse flow of current, acting instead to induce a tangential flow of current in the fluid adjacent to their surfaces. Along the surfaces of these insulating membranes, fluids flow freely. The membranes carry a negative charge. Water moves from areas of electropositive to electronegative charge. Water also accompanies positively charged ions, moving with the ions as they traverse the blood, the interstitium, and the intracellular fluids.

Ions appear in groups, according to Nordenström, because of diffusion and mechanical transport, differences in ionic mobility, influences of matrix properties, and ionic recombination. Nordenström called these ionic collections "ionars." Many investigators have studied calcium ionars for many years as stimulators of a great variety of physiological activities.[98–105] The most commonly understood calcium flux is that which is associated with the contraction of muscle. (Other examples of greater complexity are discussed later.) "The ubiquity of the calcium-oscillation is remarkable and comprises almost any eukaryotic cell so far tested" (Hess 2000, 200).

Nordenström recognized in the 1970s that ionars occur in physiological as well as pathological situations in the body. Electric circuits flowing through fluids in vessels and in the interstitium operate as basic elements of these phenomena. Although vessel walls and other fibrous constituents of the system are insulators, the capillary endothelium operates as a conductor, just like the fluids.

Lying between the nutrient capillary and the parenchymal cell, however, is the ECM, a colloid that carries a negative charge. The more negative the charge, the more stable the matrix. This stable condition represents the gel phase. A matrix with a lesser negative charge is more fluid and represents the sol phase. Calcium ionars create a strong electropositive influence, producing a sol phase in the matrix.

The calcium wave moves toward the electronegative cell membrane, taking with it a flux of water. As shifts in electric potential occur, counterions move in the opposite direction, setting up an oscillation that encourages another flux of calcium ions. Thus, we have a vital system synchronized in oscillation with respect to charge, pressure, volume, and pH. We can also measure waves of oxygen tension, nutrients, waste products, and other parameters.

In Nordenström's laboratory, electrodes showed oscillations of electrical potential in many visceral tissues to be at a rate of about 7 times per minute, the same rate as Traube and Hering measured over one hundred years earlier in vessels, and the same rate that osteopathic physicians palpate in the clinic (see Fig. 4.11).

3. Calcium Oscillations

A wave of calcium ions traveling through the matrix impacts the cell membrane and triggers intracellular calcium waves and the release of intracellular inositol triphosphate (ITP or IP_3). Further, the release of ITP produces its own modulation of free intracellular calcium ions. And, free intracellular Ca^{2+} triggers more waves of free intracellular Ca^{2+}.

Intracellular Ca^{2+} is stored in the endoplasmic reticulum, the mitochondria, and by proteins in the cytoplasm. ITP is responsible for the release of intracellular Ca^{2+} from the endoplasmic reticulum (the largest store). Mitochondria readily take in large volumes of intracellular Ca^{2+} and slowly release Ca^{2+} back into the cytosol. These various stores of Ca^{2+} interact with each other to send signals of calcium waves across the cell.[106]

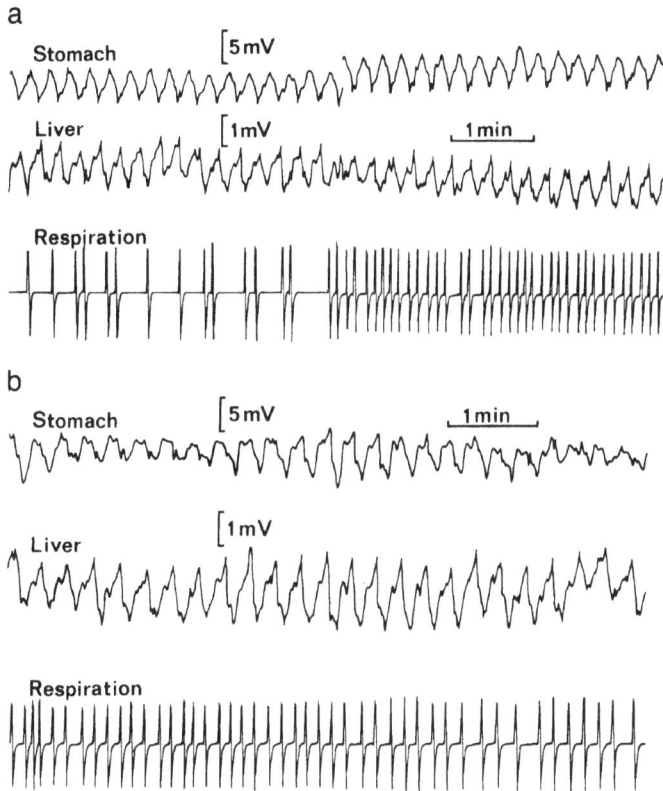

Electrical potentials from the gastric and hepatic parenchyma of a 24 kg dog . . . (a) Rhythmic fluctuations of potential from the liver. Their frequency is similar but their amplitude lower and of a slightly different pattern than that of the stomach. These rhythmic fluctuations are independent of respiration and of cardiac electrical activity. The maxima of the fluctuations of potential of the liver and the stomach varied from (a) out of phase to (b) almost in phase. Low or high amplitudes of the fluctuations of gastric potential were not accompanied by corresponding changes of amplitude in fluctuations of hepatic potential. Rhythmic fluctuations of hepatic potential have not been previously described.

4.11   Electric potentials from gastric and hepatic parenchyma. (Reproduced with permission from Nordenström BEW (1983). *Biologically Closed Electric Circuits*. Stockholm, Sweden: Nordic Medical Publications. Fig. VI:18, p. 62.)

We also know from previous discussion that cAMP triggers calcium fluxes and *vice versa*. Six mechanisms for the production of cellular calcium oscillations have been clearly identified. These involve ITP; cytoplasmic, endoplasmic reticuluar, and mitochondrial calcium; the occupied binding sites of calcium buffers; and the fraction of active ITP-receptor calcium-release channels.[107] Of course, calcium waves on the interior of the cell stimulate a variety of important and vital cellular functions.

A large body of literature elucidates the activity of calcium moving through the fluids in waves. Calcium fluxes move through the cell at a pace that is much quicker than diffusion but less rapid than axonal depolarization.[108] Four classifications of velocities of waves of calcium have been identified: ultraslow = 1–60 nm/s; slow = about 1 μm/s; fast = about 30 μm/s; and ultrafast = about 1 m/s.[109] The slow waves average about 1.5 μm/s. Because a cell measures about 15 μm, these calcium waves travel the width of a cell in about 10 seconds.

Mechanical stretching stimulates slow waves (Jaffe and Cretón, 1998). Calcium also allows increased turgor pressure to expand stretch-sensitive calcium channels in the plasma membrane (Jaffe, 1999). Thus, if flow of water is responsible for producing the stretching, calcium is both the cause and effect of increasing water and calcium movement.

E.   Matrix and Cell—The Role of Integrins

Boudreau and colleagues declare, "The extracellular matrix (ECM) profoundly influences the major programs of cell function including growth, development, and differentiation."[110] The microarchitecture of the ECM allows all the cells of the body, except the gametes and red blood cells, to fulfill their differentiated functions when interacting with the ECM structures. Cells change their phenotype in response to the extracellular environment (Rubin, 262).

The interaction of the matrix with the cell is largely through the integrins and other glycoproteins on the cell surface. Integrins, as components of the cell membrane, offer binding sites for GAGs on their amino-terminal, extracellular, *beta* subunits. The carboxy-terminal, *alpha* subunits lie inside the cell membrane and bind to vinculin, talin, and other proteins, which are called the focal adhesions of the cytoskeleton. Stimulation of the extracellular *beta* subunits of integrins activates the assemblage of focal adhesion complexes around the *alpha* subunits inside the cell. The aggregation of the focal adhesion complex stimulates outside-to-inside signaling activities from the ECM to the cytoplasm and nucleus.

Polymerization and depolymerization of the architecture of the biopolymers of the matrix have an immediate effect on the cytoskeleton by their impact on the integrins. The bonds between the GAGs and the integrins require the presence of calcium. The glycoproteins of

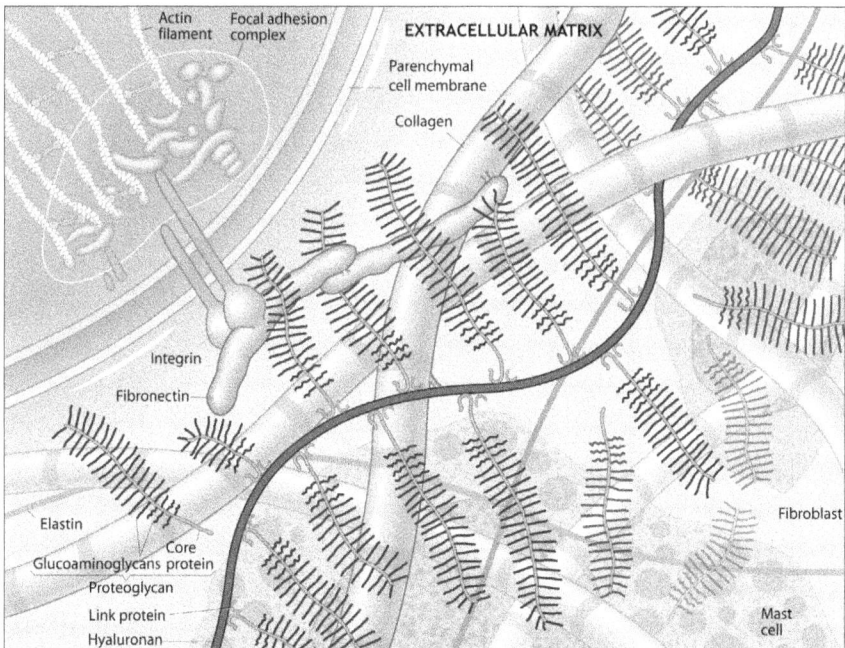

4.12   Integrins and tissue matrix. Original art by Raychel Ciemma.

the cell membrane establish their own electrical potential. A change in the potential of the matrix triggers a change in the charge of the glycoproteins of the cell membrane, which activates secondary messengers inside the cell: cAMP, cGMP, IP_3, and G proteins (Rubin, 267). G proteins activate adenylate cyclase to produce more cAMP or increase IP_3 activation of cGMP production.[111] As described earlier, these latter activities affect calcium ion flows that also trigger intracellular functions.

The intermeshing cycles of calcium ions and cAMP in the cell occurs as cAMP is secreted by the cell, hydrolyzed by phosphodiesterase, and bound to its membrane receptor with the resulting stimulation of cAMP production and desensitization of the membrane receptor.[112] Occurring at the same time is "a rapid increase in intracellular free Ca^{2+}, alkalinization of the cytosol, and phosphorylation of intracellular proteins" (Rubin, 267). In turn, this protein phosphorylation promotes adhesion of cells to ECM glycoproteins (Rubin, 273). Protein phosphorylation also seems to be important for the regulation of frequencies of intracellular calcium waves. Changes of extracellular stimuli create frequency changes of intracellular calcium fluxes with protein phosphorylation as the mediating influence (Hess 2000, 202).

F. Cell Shape and Volume

Cell shape can modulate many important cell-physiological functions such as proliferation, differentiation, and expressions of various gene products (Rubin, 262). For example, new cartilage formation is stimulated by dynamic mechanical compression, which appears to be associated mainly with changes in fluid flow, streaming potential, and/or cell shape (Grodinsky et al., 317).

Mesenchyme dictates tissue patterns when embryonic epithelia and mesenchyme are isolated from different tissues and then recombined.

For example, mixing mammary epithelium with kidney mesenchyme results in the development of tubular structures found in kidneys that secrete milk proteins. The opposite tissue mix produces shapes like breast cells that transport sodium and water.[113] When cells in culture are forced into different shapes, they can switch genetic programming. Flat cells are more likely to divide. If prevented from dividing, rounded cells activate a programmed death, apoptosis. Cells with a conformation in the middle differentiate into liver cells that secrete normal liver proteins, capillary cells that form hollow tubes, and so forth (Ingber 1998, 6).

Just, as a river maintains its shape despite a constant flow of fresh water, molecules of the living organism hold the conformation of the whole. "The molecules that make up cells and the cells that comprise tissues continually turn over: it is maintenance of pattern integrity that we call 'life' . . . Thus, a complete explanation of how cells and tissues function will come from understanding how they are put together, rather than exclusively from analysis of their substance."[114]

The maintenance of patterns, according to the hypothesis of this book, is possible because between spirit and matter there exists an *interface* composed of information from morphogenetic fields with water as the transducer and connective tissue as the receiver. This is what Still referred to by "reciprocity between the Celestial and Terrestrial."

G. Tensegrity

The Book of Nature may indeed be written in the characters of geometry. — PLATO

Buckminster Fuller first coined the term "tensegrity" from "tensional integrity" to describe the forces found in his student's architectural invention, the geodesic dome. This unique structure is self-supporting, flexible, and adaptable yet stable—qualities that also characterize living systems. Tensegrity structures apply constant tension throughout the system onto independent compressive elements. If tension increases in one place, it increases everywhere to the same degree. The global increase in tension is balanced by an increase in compression by certain members throughout the structure. Thus, the structure stabilizes itself (Ingber 1998).

In the human form, the bones are the compression elements and the tendons, muscles, and ligaments are the tension-bearing members. (Bones also provide tension within their matrix, often at right angles to compression elements.)At the other end of the scale, proteins and other key molecules stabilize through tensegrity. At any scale we wish to view, the body exhibits the same structural building blocks: spirals, pentagons, and triangles.

Looking at the gross anatomical scale, Levin[115] informs us that the spine is not a pillar of blocks transferring weight from above through the sacrum to the ilia and hips. Because volume increases cubically as the surface area of a structure squares, it is calculated that the spine would buckle from 2.2 kg of loading if weight were transferred directly down the column. Instead, the more rigid segments (bones) float in a suspensory system (ligaments), independent of gravity, with twelve degrees of freedom, each segment tensioned and/or compressed to its neighbors. If this were not the case, astronauts would explode and divers would implode from changes in pressure.

One salient example of a tensegrity structure in the human form is the sacrum. It is a hard, bony, compression element suspended between the ilia by strong, ligamentous tension elements. It can function in any posture and transfer considerable loads as a tensegrity system. These tensional and compressive forces are transmitted through straight lines because the elements are fully triangulated. In health, there are no torsional, bending, or shearing forces, only straight-line forces. Ligaments retain their constant lengths in a constant tension system as individual segments move in tandem with other segments in tension-coupled movement patterns. Compression members and tension elements retain their properties even under load. It's all share and share alike.[116]

Donald Ingber (1993) studied tensegrity in biologic systems. He realized that cellular tensegrity is just as critical to the healthy functioning of the organism as is gross myofascial tensegrity. In 1975, he first recognized that the cytoskeleton, that is, the microtubules, intermediate filaments, and actin microfilaments behave like tensegrity structures. The microtubules serve as the discontinuous compression elements and the actin microfilaments as the continuous tension elements. These two characteristics define tensegrity and qualify the cytoskeleton as a tensegrity structure. The microtubules resist compression applied by the tensioning activity of the microfilaments. Thus, the independently placed microtubules float within a sea of continuous tension from microfilaments. The whole system is stable but dynamic.

Ingber recognized that tensegrity systems display the phenomenon of self-assembly, in which components join to form larger, stable structures having properties that cannot be predicted from the characteristics of their individual parts. For example, large molecules self-assemble into organelles, which self-assemble into cells, which self-assemble into tissues, which self-assemble into organs. Of course, these principles can be found everywhere in nature. In the human, self-assembly is directed by the connective tissue elements, including the intracellular microtubules, microfilaments, and intermediate filaments. The intermediate filaments integrate the activity of the other two components. Outside the cell, the ECM exerts an essential mechanical function with the intracellular elements.

Microfilaments contain polymerized actin and sometimes myosin filaments. They are highly linear, thus exhibiting constant tension. Microtubules are hollow tubular polymers that resist bending and twisting. They are composed of tubulin monomers of various types. Sometimes microtubules exhibit buckling, indicating the axial compression that they sustain.

Intermediate filaments are composed of vimentin, desmin,

cytokeratin, and other protein monomers that are highly flexible and crenulated. These interconnect cell-cell and cell-ECM adhesion sites. They function as guy wires to stabilize the entire cytoskeletal network. This network of three types of components also suspends the nucleus in the center of the cell, and connects with the histones of the nuclear cytoskeleton. The term "tissue matrix" is applied to define a unitary mechanical function of the ECM, cell membranes, cytoskeleton, and the nuclear matrix.

The common shapes that the cytoskeleton tends to form are tetrahedrons and related shapes. One common type is the icosahedron, which Levin (1997) stated is the most economical form. It is composed of twenty equilateral triangles, thirty edges, and twelve vertices. The icosahedron can naturally be generated from the tetrahedron. The icosahedron contains the most volume per surface area of any naturally occurring form, except for the sphere, and permits a wide variety of interconnections. Pressure at any point on the surface of the icosahedron is transmitted along the thirty edges, some under tension and some under compression. It is transmitted evenly around the outer shell, as are the forces in the bicycle wheel. Pentagons are also frequently encountered, as are triangles. Pentagons are also seen in structured water; the arrangement of the water molecules around a hydrophobic element in solution forms hydrogen bonds connecting water molecules in the shape of pentagons.

Microfilaments, microtubules, and intermediate filaments respond to varying stresses on the system by remodeling, polymerizing, depolymerizing, or hardening. Nevertheless, they constantly transmit forces of tension and compression by maintaining a central core of filaments.[117] The microfilament tensegrity system is like that of muscles since it uses ATP in conjunction with actomyosin sliding to develop tension, which is responsible for changes in form (Ingber 1993).

Borrowing from the language of architecture, Ingber used the term "prestress" to characterize the tension or "tone" that the microfilaments maintain within the cell. Keeping a constant tension is also achieved by adding monomers of tubulin to microtubules if tension within the cell eases.[118] "Many of the patterns exhibited by the actin CSK [cytoskeleton] may result from dynamic remodeling of a continuous tensegrity network," determined by the microfilaments (Ingber 1993, 619). Later research showed that tugging on cell surface receptors immediately reorients the cellular components. The cell flattens, the nucleus descends to the bottom of the cell, and the organelles line up with the tension.[119] In this manner, the ECM plays an important role in tensioning the cell through membrane receptors. Integrins are a common cell membrane receptor for such mechanical stressors. Elements of the ECM attach to the integrins, as previously discussed. If integrins are experimentally twisted, the entire cell immediately stiffens, verifying the attachment of cytoskeletal elements to the integrins.[120]

H. Metabolic Consequences of Biomechanics

Has not your acquaintance with the human body opened your mind's eye to observe that in the laboratory of the human body, the most wonderful chemical results are being accomplished every day, minute and hour of your life? — A. T. STILL

Ingber's research showed that mechanical motions of elements of tensegrity have metabolic consequences. The reverse is also true—metabolic activity creates mechanical activity, a well-known feature of muscles. However, cellular metabolism requires the mechanical activity of the ECM, microfilaments, microtubules, and integrins on the cell surface. "Cells recognize and respond to mechanical stresses by changing their shape, growth, expression of specific gene products, and cytoskeletal organization, as well as by remodeling their extracellular matrix."[121] Within seconds to minutes of mechanical perturbation of the cell, several changes in activity have been measured: activation of G protein, release of chemical second messengers (e.g., arachidonic acid, cAMP, ITP, and calcium), phosphorylation of proteins, secretion of growth factors, alterations of the cytoskeleton, remodeling of cell-ECM adhesions, and changes in gene expression.[122]

In chronic mechanical stress, research has shown that once mechanical stress is removed from cells, cAMP production, arachidonic acid levels, and intracellular Ca^{2+} increase.[123] From what has been previously noted, increased cAMP and calcium levels are consistent with the healthy functioning of cells. Thus, if traumatic forces continue to produce mechanical stress in the connective tissues—as in whiplash syndrome—cell functioning is compromised. Fatigue is understandable in somatic dysfunction. The accumulation of toxins with resultant nociceptive pain is explained.

Research has shown that cell movement and growth occurs opposite to the direction of the propagation of the cAMP signal (Hess 2000, 206). The same mechanical stimulus may produce different responses, depending on the presence of various hormones or depending on which type of ECM substrate the cell is adherent to.

Mechanotransduction, the process by which mechanical energy is converted into electrical or biochemical signals, depends on three domains for its specific characteristics: extracellular, membrane, and cytoplasmic (Ingber 1997, 577). Mechanoelectric transduction operates in the neuroendocrine system at the molecular or membrane level and in the cell on a multicellular level and an organ level. It also demonstrates elements of a feedback system, interacts with other systems, and can malfunction.[124] According to studies by Wang, Butler, and Ingber (1993), mechanotransduction is essentially instantaneous throughout the whole cell and thus more rapid than diffusion.

Pienta and Coffey[125] suggested that cells transfer information through a system that they called the tissue matrix (see Fig. 4.14). They defined the tissue matrix as the extracellular matrix, the cytoskeleton, and the nuclear matrix down to the DNA. They asserted that the tissue matrix system may transfer information and direct cell structure and function in a dynamic tensegrity-matrix structure. Through the tensegrity system, information is transferred from the cell periphery through the cytoplasm and into the nuclear matrix system that organizes the chromatin and DNA. This transfer of information can occur through harmonic wave motions that are propagated along a tensor within the matrix. Information passed through the tensor depends in part on the amplitude and frequency of the wave propagating along it. One theory states that the amount of information that a tensor system can pass is equal to the width of the frequency band of the waves of information and the total time they are available for interpretation. The quick and directed flow of vibrational information is transmitted both in series and parallel by using the branching network of the cell matrix.

Pienta and Coffey reported various frequencies of cellular component oscillations.

- DNA ranges in vibrations from 10^{-11} to 10^{-12} second.

- Protein oscillates from 10^{-12} to 1 second.

- Ion fluxes oscillate from 0.4 to 100 seconds.

- Membranes produce ruffling in oscillations lasting 6–60 seconds.

- Membranes undulate at rates of 6–15 minutes.

- Cell cycles of growth, cell division, and stable metabolic activity occur every 18–48 hours.

Of course, palpable oscillations are of special interest to osteopathic physicians, making the ion fluxes of special interest. Calcium fluxes, as we have already seen, fulfill the criteria as agents of information transfer that could be palpable, their oscillations occurring in the frequency range of the primary respiratory mechanism.

Pienta and Coffee went on to say that the frequencies of cellular

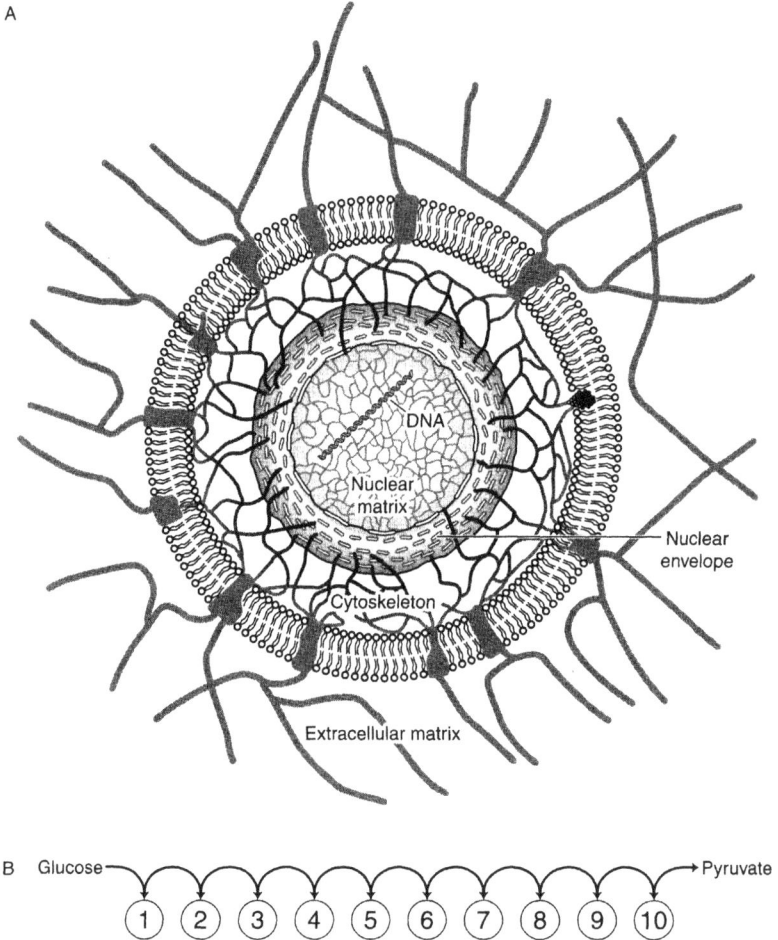

(A) Contemporary image of a cell and its relations: the living matrix. Modern cell biology has recognized that the cell interior is virtually filled with fibers and tubes and filaments, collectively called the cytoskeleton or cytoplasmic matrix. Likewise, the nucleus contains a nuclear matrix that supports the genetic material. Linkers called integrins extend across the cell surface, connecting the cytoskeleton with the extracellular matrix. The entire system is termed the living matrix.

(B) Shows a more realistic model of a biochemical pathway, glycolysis, in which the enzymes are organized in sequence along the cytoskeletal structure. The reaction sequence can proceed very rapidly because reactants are passed from one enzyme to the next to the next, as in an assembly line.

4.13 Tissue matrix. (Reproduced from Oschman JL (2000). *Energy Medicine.* New York: Churchill Livingstone. Fig. 3.2, p. 46. Reprinted with permission from Elsevier Inc.)

vibrations might be tuned by their contacts with the tensegrity matrix as well as by varying tensions that are controlled through the energy metabolism of the cell. The energy metabolism is modified by cell-signaling processes such as calcium, protein kinase C, guanine nucleotide-binding proteins, and inositol phosphates. These elements of cell signaling are recognized as cytoskeletal components. Enzyme cascades require spatial and temporal patterning for activation. Such timing and location of enzymes are best accomplished by the tissue matrix system, which also modifies the tension component (i.e., actin) and the polymerization of the compression elements (i.e., microtubules) of the cytoskeleton. Thus, the cell is hardwired in a structure-function relationship as part of the tissue matrix system (Pienta and Coffey 1991).

Ingber and Jamieson[126] suggested that architectural variations in the tissue matrix system can result in local pressure and volume changes, which in turn can alter the free energy available for activation of enzyme systems. The dynamic state of the tissue tensegrity matrix

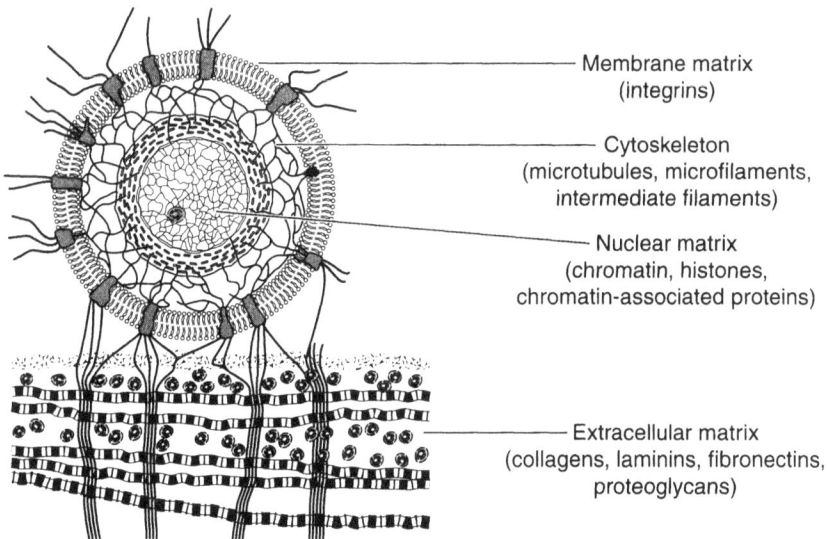

4.14 Tissue matrix system as described by Pienta and Coffey, 1991. (Reproduced from Oschman JL (2000). *Energy Medicine.* New York: Churchill Livingstone. Fig. 4.6, p. 66. Reprinted with permission from Elsevier Inc. and Medical Hypotheses.)

uses harmonic, particulate, thermodynamic, and soluble signals for the modulation of its architecture. The microtubules, microfilaments, and intermediate filaments each provide unique mechanical functions to transmit particulate information among the peripheral, cytosolic, and nuclear compartments (Pienta and Coffey 1991). We previously noted that research by Vern and Biswal demonstrated that certain functions of the body increase metabolic activity in specific regions of the brain, which is also associated with increased fluid and mechanical activity there (see Section III.C.5: "Metabolic Rhythms").

Cytoskeletal tension, determined by the sliding of the actomyosin of the microfilaments, is the major force acting on living cells, and all external loads impose themselves on a preexisting cytoskeletal force (Ingber 1997). One of the important effects of intracellular calcium waves is to change the conformation of the cytoskeleton by causing a contraction of the actomyosin filaments. Calcium waves also stimulate the activity of enzymes that are bound to the cytoskeleton, perhaps by approximating adjacent microtubules and their attached enzymes. The enzymes are carefully ordered on the microtubule structure to maximize efficient functioning of the chain of reactions without having to cast the substrate and product out into solution after each biochemical reaction. Instead, the substrate and product are held by the system of cytoskeleton and enzymes and passed along, one enzyme to the next, in the process of the substrate's degradation or synthesis. In fact, there is very little water available in which any substrate, product, or other substance might be dissolved. Even though there is ubiquitous water in the cell, it is mostly bound to cellular constituents and behaves differently than water that is free and unbound. This function of transferring one enzymatic product to the next enzyme as its substrate without equilibrating with bulk solution is termed metabolic channeling. Further, microcompartmentation of metabolites segregates labile intermediates from competing reactions, affording an efficient and rapid biochemical outcome.[127]Assembly-line like chains of enzymes are called metabolons.

"Much of the cell's machinery functions in a solid state" (Ingber 1997, 588). As early as 1940, Sherrington recognized the ordered nature of the cell's interior. He said, "Although it is fluid and watery, most of the cell is not a true solution. A drop of true solution, of homogeneous liquid, could not 'live'. It is remote from 'organization'. In the cell there are heterogeneous solutions. The great molecules of protein and aggregated particles are suspended not dissolved. A surface is field for chemical and physical action. The interior of a pure solution has no surfaces. But the aggregate of surface of these foamy colloids which are in the cell mounts up to something large. The 'internal surface' of the cell is enormous. The cell gives chemical results which in the laboratory are obtained only by temperatures and pressures far in excess of those in the living body. Part of the secret of life is the immense internal surface of the cell."[128]

More recently, a number of investigators described this crucial relationship between the internal structure of the cell and its function. Ingber noted that the biochemical reactions of protein synthesis, RNA transport, glycolysis, and DNA synthesis all appear to involve the channeling of sequestered substrates and products from one fixed enzyme to another along cytoskeletal filaments. For example, mRNAs specifically localize to intersections between different actin filaments rather than along their length. Thus, architectural changes—triangulated nets to linear bundles—of the cytoskeleton from stresses applied to the tensegrity system could influence protein synthesis (Ingber 1997). J. Clegg pointed out that changing the relative position of specific regulatory molecules alters their ability to chemically interact.[129] It is known that alterations in enzyme activity occur by alterations in their biophysical conformation and flexibility. Thus, under the influence of the tissue matrix system, mechanical energy is transformed directly into chemical energy.[130] Therefore, touch affects metabolism.

Glycolysis is a salient example of enzyme systems being bound to cytoskeletal elements. The activity of these enzymes oscillates. Glycolytic enzymes are more active when bound to cytoskeletal elements than when unbound (Al-Habori 1995, 128). The binding of enzymes to the cytoskeleton is characterized by low binding energies, implying that they exist in equilibrium between bound and unbound states. Various influences impinge on this system to establish and alter the rates of the cycles of ATP production. The concentration of metabolic factors, pH, and the presence of hormones changes the dynamics of the system.

Insulin, epinephrine, and glucagon increase the binding of glycolytic enzymes to the cytoskeleton. These hormones also increase the polymerization of actin microfilaments. Any perturbation of cell surface receptors increases the production of actin as well. Calcium stimulates the contraction of these actin filaments, thus drawing reactants into microcompartments and producing more ATP. Simultaneously, increased intracellular Ca^{2+} and intracellular cAMP both stimulate glycolysis.[131] And cAMP and Ca^{2+} positively promote the increased concentration of the other. All of these influences on metabolism create a feed-forward stimulus to increase the production of ATP that is initiated by calcium waves in the extracellular compartment.

Glycogen synthesis, on the other hand, involves the reverse of actin contraction, that is, cell swelling. Insulin stimulates an increase of cell volume and glycogen synthesis. Al-Habori (1995) postulated that cell swelling is responsible for organizing the cytoskeleton, which in turn activates the enzymes that synthesize glycogen. Thus, we can see how contraction and swelling of the cell are two differing actions associated with two different cellular functions. Cell contraction is related to glycolysis and the production of ATP, while cell swelling is related to glycogen synthesis and the utilization of ATP. Thus, we see that the oscillation of cell volume produced by calcium waves in the extracellular matrix initiates and regulates the basic energy metabolism of the cell by changing the architecture of the cytoskeleton.

It was shown in 1977 that large fluorescent-tagged protein molecules move to all parts of the cell in 1 second.[132] This is far too fast for simple diffusion. Wheatley postulated in 1985, before cell oscillations were well documented, that two possibilities existed to explain the movement of nutrients inside the solid-state cell. One explanation was random movements, assisted by the ebb-and-flow movements from the overall activity of the cell. This is analogous to the popular concept about the movement of blood before Harvey discovered its one-way circulation. The other possibility for this rapid distribution of large molecules inside the cell was an organized movement of "cytocirculation" occurring in defined, if labile and transient, channels describing a unidirectional pathway.[133]

Those who palpate the oscillation of the tissues might opt for Wheatley's first possibility because they understand by *prima fasciae* palpatory evidence that there is an ebb-and-flow in the tissues. Wheatley made the case, however, for cytoplasmic streaming, the second possibility, as the means by which large proteins move rapidly through the cell. Measurements of the time it takes for similar proteins to move through various media over similar distances *in vitro*, are 20–30 times longer than *in vivo*, Wheatley said. He asserted that an organized movement system operates at high speeds in living systems, but he did not rule out an ebb-and-flow mechanism. He said, "A common distribution system bringing in essential nutrients and removing waste products would therefore seem to be a reasonable proposition at the cellular level, just as our blood circulatory system operates effectively to supply our entire body" (Wheatley 1985, 306). Thus, the movement of nutrients and waste products within the cell respond to an energy-consuming system, such as that predicted by W. G. Sutherland, DO, not passive diffusion. It is the contention of this author that Sutherland was correct in his hypothesis that an ebb-and-flow mechanism supplies the nutrients to the cells. Once the capillaries deliver oxygen and glucose, for example, to the ECM by a circulatory stream, an ebb-and-flow mechanism takes over to transport the nutritional elements to the cell surface and within the cell itself.

Cooper (1995, 77) postulated that cells secrete solutes by cyclical mechanisms. Cycles are regulated by a series of events. Cells steadily absorb solutes and their osmotically associated water from the extracellular space. Their cell membranes become distended.[134–135] With the distention of cell membranes, stretch-activated ion channels that are permeable to Ca^{2+} are activated to a critical point. Extracellular Ca^{2+} enters the cell through such stretch-activated channels. This causes calcium-activated potassium channels to open, resulting in a rapid efflux of potassium out of the cell. As KCl leaves the cell, water follows osmotically, resulting in a decrease in cell volume.

In addition to stretch-activated volume regulation, calcium also regulates cell volume through phosphatidyl-inositol metabolism in pancreatic acinar cells in which periodic potassium-water secretion decreases cell volume.[136] Kasai and Augustine proposed that a polarization of cytosolic Ca^{2+} elevation and ion channel activation actively propel ions and their osmotically associated water in a unidirectional manner through secretory cells.[137] Further, Cooper (1995, 79) postulated that visible contractions *in vivo* and *in vitro* of glial cells correspond to the measured cyclical efflux of solutes and water. He proposed that these activities are under the control of Ca^{2+}-calmodulin through its influence on myosin light-chain kinase, which causes the contraction of the cytoskeletal (CSK) actin microfilaments.

In 1985, Foskett and Spring[138] reported that cell volume increase is independent from interstitial calcium but that volume contraction depends on calcium stimulation of actin microfilaments. In 1989, Foskett and Melvin[139] reported in *Science* that intracellular calcium levels correspond to cell volume. In physiological ranges, increasing intracellular Ca^{2+} causes cell volume to shrink. They noted that cell volume corresponds linearly with intracellular Ca^{2+}, even with calcium oscillations. Further, they were able to show that solutes move into and out of the cell with these modulations of intracellular Ca^{2+}. For these effects to persist, it was necessary to have physiological concentrations of extracellular Ca^{2+}.

Schwab et al.[140]determined that the Ca^{2+}-sensitive K^+ channel is activated by cell shrinkage and inhibited by cell swelling. Further, cell shrinkage induces a slight decrease in intracellular Ca^{2+}, and cell swelling induces an increase in intracellular Ca^{2+}. The latter influences bring the calcium concentrations back into balance and tend to instigate calcium waves. Kizer et al.[141] reported that cell swelling induces membrane depolarization, which is accompanied by a transient increase in intracellular Ca^{2+}. Light et al.[142] determined that cell swelling led to ATP efflux from the cell, which stimulated calcium-dependant cell shrinkage and K^+ efflux. Marunaka et al.[143] showed that, in the presence of Ca^{2+}, insulin increased cell volume and, in the absence of Ca^{2+}, insulin induced cell shrinkage. All of these findings support the hypothesis that calcium ion concentration is involved in producing cyclical cell-volume changes and solute movement into and out of the cell.

Al-Habori[144] pointed out that "At the cellular level, insulin controls ion transport, glucose and substrate uptake (e.g., amino acids) as well as the phosphorylation and dephosphorylation of enzymes." Further, insulin affects the cytoskeleton and changes cell volume. It seems to accomplish this effect by increasing the intracellular K^+ without exchanging the flow of K^+ to the interior of the cell with other ions to the exterior. This net increase in cationic content in the cell creates an osmotic increase in cell volume.

These research results lead us to the conclusion that the cycles of water flowing into and out of the cells depend on hormones, ions, and the condition of the extracellular matrix. The interrelationships of all these factors—calcium ion concentration, hormone levels, and flow of potassium and calcium ions, as well as the other previously mentioned influences of water binding, electrostatic charge, hydrogen bonding, hydrophobic forces, flows of electrons, approximation of enzymes within the cells, and stimulation of chromosomal DNA—create interlocking mechanisms of cycles of activity.

The details of these individual activities, when taken together, support the contention of this book that there are biochemical explanations for the palpatory experience of the clinician. The primary respiratory mechanism is a well-orchestrated system down to the subcellular, molecular, and energetic level of mechanotransduction, involving the entire tissue matrix system. The tissue matrix system, including the ECM, the cytoskeleton, and the nuclear matrix, works together as one unit effecting the chemical and mechanical changes of metabolic activity. Cell function depends on extracellular function. Self-healing depends on these biochemical mechanisms. Whatever therapy is employed, these same mechanisms manifest whatever healing we observe. These molecular mechanisms operate as a unit of function, demonstrate the interrelationship of structure and function (mechanotransduction), and describe the manner in which the body heals itself.

V. INTERFACE: FORM AND MOTION

In this chapter, I have presented philosophical and scientific information to support the contention that as osteopathic physicians we palpate the essence of life, on which Dr. Still based his philosophy. We work with the interface between the Celestial and Terrestrial. We experience the whole as we touch the patient and engage the holographic connective tissue and the movement that plies it. Underlying all we do is the emergence of Health, which manifests as the primary respiratory mechanism. Health comes from the perfection of the universe into that which has been distorted. Palpating the primary respiratory mechanism, we access spirit coming into form. At this interface, healing happens.

No matter what intention, technique, medication, or surgical procedure we might employ, Health does the work of healing. The primary respiratory mechanism, through the transformation at still point, performs the healing that permits the continuation of spirit in physical manifestation. The original form is restored through changing the physical form to match the energetic blueprint; distortion is able to return to the original form. The energy of spirit operates the machine that Dr. Still envisioned. It moves the calcium ions to recharge and de-polymerize the matrix. The ions stimulate the cells, distending them with the accompanying water, and invigorating them with the accompanying nutrients. The activities of life continue.

Grossly palpable motion derives from these miniscule operations. The mechanisms for such phenomena are ubiquitous. Everywhere that science explores, it finds motion. Life is motion. All we need to do as physicians is to see that spirit's urge to move is restored. Then, health returns.

5

INTERFACE:

AN OSTEOPATHIC PERSPECTIVE

The little things are infinitely the most important.
— SIR ARTHUR CONAN DOYLE

Frrom the founder of osteopathic medicine, Andrew Taylor Still, MD, DO, we receive the notion that creation is based on Mind, Matter, and Motion. Mind (Celestial) reciprocates with Matter (Terrestrial) to produce Motion (Life). The model presented in this book describes the interface of this reciprocity. William Garner Sutherland, DO, Still's student, described this interface more fully when he discovered and elucidated the primary respiratory mechanism. He indicated that the primary respiratory mechanism exhibits the life force to which Dr. Still referred as the product of the reciprocity between the Celestial and Terrestrial. Sutherland taught that the primary respiratory mechanism manifested from the Breath of Life. He believed that this subtle inherent motion in the tissues was an exposition of spirit, another word for his breath of life. For Still, the life force or Unconditional Love is the very ground substance of all creation. The thesis of this book declares that, when we palpate the primary respiratory mechanism, we are palpating the effects of this fundamental force of the universe. Up to this point, this unseen profound power of living organisms has not been explained in scientific terms. As a fundamental precept of osteopathic philosophy from Still, this mechanism of reciprocity deserves full elucidation.

This book draws together many resources to explain the functions of the cell and the connective tissue relative to the life force. It looks at both the spiritual and biochemical realities of the primary respiratory mechanism that we are acquainted with in the clinical setting as a palpatory phenomenon. The model explains for me how the life force, which underlies all osteopathic philosophy, interfaces with the material aspect, creating evidence of life and health. The model characterizes Motion interfacing between Mind and Matter. Motion is life. Mind, Matter, and Motion are all aspects of spirit, but Motion—life—is the special characteristic that produces the tide, which delivers health in an otherwise nonliving body of connective tissue. The breath of life is a motionless ever-present influence in the realm of spirit that manifests in the physical realm as a fluctuation that is palpable.

Spirit, in the context of this book, is a phenomenological reality with an explicit purpose when considering material manifestations. Spirit develops mechanisms for its impulse to exist in physical reality. These mechanisms are deployed through various physical means—revealed through biochemistry and cellular physiology, among other disciplines—for spirit to be housed in a physical body.

The structural pattern of the life form exists in an energetic spiritual realm and relates to the physical realm through the media of water, electricity, and probably other yet-to-be-identified subtle influences. A pattern of charge—the morphogenetic field—in the energy realm organizes the charged elements of the connective tissue that, in a watery medium, establishes a physical form in which all organs and functions find their home.

Functions (in the implicate order) precede the structure. The structure (in the explicate order) accommodates the function. However, once established, the structure rules the maintenance of the function. If the structure is distorted, the function cannot operate at its optimum.

Reestablishing the conformation of the original structure to harmonize with the original morphogenetic field allows the reestablishment of healthy function. This is the purpose of osteopathic manipulative treatment—to permit health to reemerge.

There is also the matter of self-assembly, in which structure arises out of the intrinsic nature of the structural components, without any apparent influence from function. Much embryological assembly occurs according to this process, as Blechschmidt showed so eloquently.[1] The means for building organisms through self-assembly does not detract from the function-leads-to-structure argument, however. Spirit efficiently uses established patterns in the physical world for its purposes. The success of one pattern can be used again to advance form and function as life moves to higher and higher expressions of spirit. For example, the success of unicellular creatures can be employed in creating aggregates of cells—multicellular creatures. Such an enormous step in the advancement of life forms demands another function—integrating cells into unitary action that is good for the whole. Connective tissue serves this function; yet these tissues self-assemble, facilitating spirit's impulse to progress.

Self-assembly is an ongoing process in the maintenance of health. When we use a therapeutic modality, such as osteopathic manipulative treatment, the body may apply the energy that takes the organism toward greater balance to self-assemble more microtubules for cellular reshaping as the stress of the tissue matrix system is relieved. No matter which osteopathic technique is employed, the health is restored from within. The tide delivers the health through the medium of water, electrolytes, and other solutes. The perfection of the structural pattern, established by a morphogenetic field, originally displays a perfection of function. With trauma, imperfection of the structural element displays imperfection of function. If we refer to the perfection of the original pattern, both structure and function resume their original perfection. The structural aspect is that which is disturbed and therefore must be corrected; the spiritual pattern retains its perfection. Matching this perfection, with manipulation of the physical, restores the physical disturbance to balance and allows the urge of the spiritual to emerge in its perfection. By this means, health moves. In the tissues, we palpate health as a full and symmetric tide. Peace, harmony, happiness, and balance are outward signs of health in the behavior and demeanor of the individual.

Distortions of the energetic aspect also occur through emotion, thought, and behavior that are not harmonious with balance, health, and love. These energetic influences perturb function as much as physical influences. We usually consider these disturbances of health to be in the realm of psychology and not treatable by osteopathic approaches. There is an opportunity here for the application of osteopathic philosophy and practice as presented in this model to rebalance the body's energy, although such an approach has not been specifically addressed in this writing. We could offer energetic treatment from an osteopathic perspective, but this dimension of health care deserves a separate writing.

What are the biochemical characteristics of the tide that we palpate in the body? Water mediates the transmission of the impetus for physical life. Calcium ions carry the message in the water as a specific trigger for many functions. In the interstitium, when waves of calcium ions pass through, the normal gel phase dissolves into a sol phase, permitting nutrients and waste products to flow through. The fibrous constituents of the extracellular matrix (ECM) depolymerize with the increased concentrations of calcium ions. With depolymerization of the ground substance, water that is bound to the negatively charged domains of the glucoaminoglycans (GAGs) becomes unbound and flows with the charged calcium ions.

Water accompanying the wave of calcium ions moves the dissolved glucose, oxygen, and hormones from the nutrient capillary to the parenchymal cell much more quickly than diffusion can. Receptors on the surface of the cells receive these stimuli to enact metabolic functions within the cell.

Through the integrins on the cell membrane, the microfilaments of the cytoskeleton contract with the stimulus of the calcium wave on the cell surface, approximating microtubules and microfilaments inside the cell, activating enzyme systems, and forcing water and waste products out of the cell. The waste products flow, during this sol phase of the ECM, into the venous capillaries and the open fenestrations of the neighboring lymphatic channels.

The concentration of free water outside the cell increases, driving the free water into the venous and lymphatic capillaries and the cells. As the concentration of free water reaches a maximum, the calcium ion concentration reaches a minimum and the ECM repolymerizes, recreating a gel phase.

In the gel phase of the ECM, the fenestrations of the lymph vessels close, trapping waste products and water in the lymphatic capillaries. Nutrients flow into the cell with the flow of free water as the cell swells. Enzyme systems that were activated in the cell contraction (at the beginning of the sol phase of the ECM) are deactivated, while other enzyme systems are activated in the swelling phase of the cell.

Nutrients, as information, create their own stimuli, even to the nuclear genetic material. Certain DNA might be stimulated, while other strands are folded and deactivated. Mitochondria take up water, oxygen, and glucose, waiting for the next cell contraction to expel carbon dioxide and water into the cytoplasm.

Meanwhile, in the ECM, charged particles such as hydrogen ions or other counterions have flowed in the opposite direction of the previous calcium wave to reset the potential and to generate another wave of calcium ions. The cell membrane is comparatively negatively charged relative to the surrounding ECM, attracting the positively charged calcium ions.

All of these individual activities exist in the cell and ECM and have been scientifically documented, studied, and elucidated. They simply have not been integrated into a single model of an oscillatory motion as depicted here. We know that such an oscillatory motion exists by *prima facie* evidence. The individual elements of this model have been scientifically worked out, but they come to us as information. The integration of these elements into a unified model derives from clinical palpatory knowledge.

As an example, we know that water flows in a river from *prima facie* evidence, or knowledge. If I stand in the river, I feel the pressure of the water on my body that gives me that knowledge firsthand. We also know that water behaves biochemically in certain way—for example as structured water—from scientific research, or information. If I read instruments under well-controlled circumstances, I conclude, secondhand, that water exhibits a certain pH, oxygen tension, and resistivity.

The integration of firsthand and secondhand experiences is a valid method to further our understanding of the world. However, we do not want to make the mistake of discounting knowledge that is not measured secondhand by instruments when we can feel it firsthand. We do not want to make the mistake of discounting reality simply because we cannot find it on the map. One day, the map will be completed to describe what we already know exists in reality.

This is where clinicians have the advantage over bench scientists, who want to be able to demonstrate reality by some secondhand means of measurement. The model presented here assumes that the oscillation of the tide exists and merely seeks a scientific explanation of it. The elements of the oscillation have all been proven. The model is a hypothesis to draw all the elements together into one reasonable explanation.

This explanation creates a model that incorporates the idea that the macromolecular structure of the cell and the ECM is highly organized and that its function is likewise well ordered. The detailed structure of the cytoskeleton and the extracellular matrix begs for a mechanism to explain it. Of course, the reverse is also true. For those of us who feel the primary respiratory mechanism, we find the explanation for it exists in the highly ordered macromolecular structure and function.

Once we believed that the cell was a bag of soup, and that the ECM was amorphous. Now we understand that enzymes work in a solid state rather than in solution. They are attached to and ordered in sequence along elements of the cytoskeleton. Mechanical energy approximates and separates tubules and microfilaments to activate and deactivate these enzymes, transducing biomechanical and biochemical energy.

The contraction of the cytoskeletal microfilaments with an efflux of free water or swelling of the cell with an influx of free water provides the means to accomplish the approximation or disengagement. ATP supplies the power for these actions, and calcium ions or cAMP supply the stimulus to produce the ATP.

The ECM dissolves to permit the fuel for the production of ATP—glucose—to cross the no-man's land of the interstitium and enter the cell. All these actions involve the expenditure of biomechanical and bioelectrical energy. Biodynamics, the transformation between biomechanical and bioelectrical energy is an essential aspect of the activities of life.

Further, the hard wiring of the tissue matrix system makes a continuous fibrous network of connective tissue elements from the subcutaneous tissue to the ECM, cytoskeleton, nucleus, and genes. Touching the surface of the skin, we are able to access all parts of the body through the connective tissue network—the tissue matrix.

We work holistically when we work with the holographic connective tissue. Mechanical activity accompanies electrical activity within the tissue matrix system. Applying a mechanical stimulus to the surface of the skin affects the electrical activity throughout the system.

Further, there is no single place, no fundamental aspect, and no primary part of the living matrix. The properties of the whole network depend on the integrated activities of all the components. Effects on one part can, and do, affect the rest.

This is a vital image of the living structure of the body. Our images shape our therapeutic success. These images give rise to intentions, and intentions give rise to electrical and magnetic activities in the central nervous system (CNS) of the operator. These patterns of energy can influence the body of the patient.

Working with the primary respiratory mechanism, Sutherland instructed us that we can effect healing. He indicated that, when the oscillation comes to stillness, there is an exchange among all fluid compartments in the organism. With this fluid exchange comes a transmutation. A transmutation—a change in the constituents, character, or nature of the fluids—is the means by which the potency expresses the new condition of the treated tissues. If we accept his pronouncements about these fluid movements and transmutations as *prima facie* details of reality, we might desire a further biochemical explanation.

I propose that during a still point, transmutation expresses itself when, momentarily, intracellular and extracellular compartments simultaneously exist in a sol state. The free exchange of water, solutes, and information among all systems is permitted. It is like pushing the metabolic reset button; the entire organism is open. This occurs in a fashion similar to the experiment performed during a complete solar eclipse, in which water was shaken as it received the sun's energy according to the progression of the eclipse—full sun, partial sun, or no sun. Later, wheat germinated according to the amount of sunlight that the water had received as it was shaken (see Chapter Four, Section III. C.4: "Water's Sensitivity Receives Life"). The openness of the water was maximized by the shaking. The openness allowed a transformation in the water; and the water passed on to the wheat seedlings the information it received while it was open. This is the idea of what happens when the whole body achieves a still point. Information is transmitted throughout because of its openness. The still point offers a reference point to the originality of the morphogenetic field.

I further propose that Sutherland's cranial concept can be summarized in an expanded way. His original concept included the following five elements, to which we can add a sixth.

1. Inherent motility of the central nervous system.
2. Fluctuation of the cerebrospinal fluid.
3. Mobility of the intracranial and intraspinal dural membranes.
4. Mobility of the cranial bones.
5. Mobility of the sacrum between the ilia.
6. These five effects upon the rest of the system.

In proposing this expanded summary, I intend to generalize the cranial concept to include the entire body. Beyond the fluctuation of the CSF, all interstitial fluids of the body fluctuate. In fact, fluctuation of intracellular fluids is responsible for the inherent motion of the cells. Rather than the brain alone having inherent motion, all the organs of the body bear this characteristic. Likewise, all connective tissues, not just the dural membranes of the CNS, through their piezoelectric and tensegrity qualities, integrate and coordinate fluid activities. Instead of cranial bone motion, we can generalize to say all bones in the body have oscillatory motion.

Next, I propose that we can distill the original five elements into two general statements that represent the two elements that reciprocate, according to Still: spirit and matter. According to the model proposed here, the inherent motion of the CNS and the fluctuation of the CSF are part of the same process. This process reflects the activity of spirit. Thus, we can conclude that the breath of life results in the motions of the ions and water in the interstitium and cells associated with an organized swelling and receding of the cell volume of the CNS. Simultaneously, the CSF fluctuates in reciprocal fashion.

These first two elements of the original cranial concept can be summarized as follows:

1. A palpable oscillation of the CNS occurs with the fluctuation of electrolytes and water between the intracellular and extracellular compartments.

The next three elements of Sutherland's original cranial concept—motion of the membranes, the cranial bones, and the sacrum—reflect the reciprocity of the material aspect, the connective tissues, in response to the activity of spirit through the medium of water. These elements can be summarized as follows:

2. Accommodation for this primary initiative occurs with passive motion of the cranial bones, the sacrum, and the reciprocating dural membranes, the latter serving to integrate all motions of the bones surrounding the CNS.

To generalize these two precepts to the whole body, we can say the following:

1. The movement of water and electrolytes creates alternating sol

and gel phases of the ECM that coincide with contraction and swelling phases, respectively, of the parenchymal cells and delivers nutrients and removes waste products appropriately as the basis for metabolism.

2. The connective tissues display the characteristics of piezoelectricity and tensegrity as the means by which they biomechanically, biochemically, and bioelectrically accommodate and participate in oscillating fluid metabolism.

Item 1 of this model represents spirit. Item 2 represents matter. The reciprocation of the two represents the basis of osteopathic thought. This is the *interface* in simple terms.

The following scenario is theoretical but plausible. The CNS is a special case of this fluctuant phenomenon. The CNS fluctuation orders the rest. The calcium ion and hydrogen counterion waves transduce the life force into metabolic and biomechanical activity. The generated motion is integrated throughout the CNS by the glial cells the most numerous in the brain. There are multiple intercellular bridges providing nearly instantaneous communication among glial cells, via calcium fluxes. This motion recapitulates the embryonic ram's-horn development and creates a dynamo, charging the posterior brain positively and the anterior brain negatively. The CSF derives its potency from this dynamo. The charge of the CNS, a vibrant standing wave, intensifies and subsides in cycles with this rhythmic movement. The rhythmic intensification affects not only the glial cells, but also the Schwann cells of the peripheral nerves. This is what Still referred to as "watering the withering fields."

Because the autonomic nerves end in the ECM in all tissues of the body, the waves of potency from the respiratory activity of the CNS are transmitted everywhere in the organism via the Schwann cells covering the peripheral nerves. Consequently, at the endings of the ubiquitous sympathetic nerves, norepinephrine is rhythmically released, producing a cyclical acidic effect. Acidic ECM is a gel with bound water. Increased hydrogen ion concentration in the form of a flow of counterions stimulates the opposite flow of calcium ions in the ECM. The calcium wave and its accompanying water and dissolved nutrients stimulate metabolic activity of the parenchymal cells of the entire body.

The ultimate point is that this model represents a cogent biochemical explanation of a clinical phenomenon—the primary respiratory mechanism—which is at the root of osteopathic philosophy, that is, spirit as it reveals itself in material manifestation, through reciprocity.

The spiritual component (Mind; the breath of life) reciprocates with the material component (Matter; the connective tissues, including the tissue matrix system) through the energetic component (Motion; movement of water, electrolytes, and other physiologically active molecules) to produce a life form and to maintain it via a palpable delivery of health.

The interface between matter and energy, the material and spiritual, that Still and Sutherland referred to is everywhere, if we simply look for it. It is seen in a living organism or biogen, as described by Still. The primary respiratory mechanism that Sutherland described represents the *interface*. It manifests as the very action of reciprocity that Still said is necessary to form biogen. He said that life is the most powerful force in the universe. Life engages the material elements to produce an organism in form and function.

Generative forces in the embryo are retained throughout life as healing forces. In the embryo, the morphogenetic field directs the migration of tissue to organize the organism. In the adult, healing recapitulates the development process. Migrating cells in the embryo establish the pattern for the movement of energy, the delivery of water and nutrients. The removal of waste travels in the opposite direction. This to and fro motion is palpable. It represents the reciprocity described by Still.

Consciousness underlies everything. It is the backdrop for patterns of energy that serve as the template for physical form. Physical form, on the other end of the reciprocation, needs the energetic pattern as expressed through the process of development in order to create a viable organism. Once the life force introduces itself into the mix of disorganized material and energetic elements, development and health are the result. As osteopathic physicians, we can work with the health and promote wellness, vigor, and originality. This is the highest goal of osteopathic medicine, expressed as caring, holism, and prevention.

Whether or not an individual osteopathic physician engages the primary respiratory mechanism or does any manipulation at all, he or she can express the philosophy derived from the reciprocity between Matter and Mind by demonstrating in his or her approach to practice the exquisite beauty and spiritual harmony of the organism and recognize as Drew Still did that it issues from the ultimate creative potential.

POSTSCRIPT

A. T. Still departed from the usual and customary practice of medicine after ten years of reflection on the large questions of nature and on the minute details of the perfection of the structure of the human organism. His departure left for us an example of a process we could all choose to take: distancing ourselves from old habits. He invited us to explore with him to discover the truths of Osteopathy. He said that he had only grasped the tail of the squirrel in the hole in the tree. It is for all of us to extricate the body of the squirrel from its hiding place. In 1896 he said: "Osteopathy is a science; not what we know of it, but the subject we are studying, is as deep as eternity. We know but little of it. I have worked and worried here in Kirksville for twenty-two long years, and I intend to study for twenty-three thousand years yet."[1]

He believed that Osteopathy is synonymous with truth and that it would gradually unfold and develop (Booth, 63). The author hopes that the contents of this book contribute to the greater unfolding of this truth.

The change is occurring with or without the leadership or participation of the osteopathic profession. Can the profession rediscover its past to inherit its future? After all, what if osteopathic medicine should die? What if no one remembered how to teach what Still taught? What if the edifice on Ontario Street in downtown Chicago fell silent and empty?

But wait! Healing, spirit, life, renewal are all here! They do not leave with the demise of an organization. The squirrel is still there in the hole in the tree waiting to be fully extricated. The promise of Osteopathy lives. Truth remains free. Still's voice, clear as it was, is now joined by a choir. My joy is to hear the harmonies when we all sing together.

APPENDIX

A New Understanding of A. T. Still's Philosophy

The following elements suggest the basis for a new understanding of A. T. Still's philosophy:

1. **Unconditional Love** exists as the fundamental Principle of Creation. Unconditional Love underlies and interpenetrates all energy and matter. It is all-knowing, ever-present, and all-powerful. Still characterized this principle as the Love of God. Danté and Swedenborg used similar terms to describe this universal essence.

2. The **Life Force**, which Still called spirit or life, arises within the Principle of Creation, the Celestial realm (Still) or the implicate order (Bohm). Sutherland used the term the breath of life to describe the life force. Motion, the effect of spirit in the physical realm, provides evidence for the life force, which is otherwise hidden in the energetic realm. Motion is overt evidence of the still, creative impulse.

3. **Consciousness,** which Still called Mind, also arises within the Principle of Creation and contributes awareness to creation. Mind and spirit both originate in the Celestial realm (Still) or implicate order (Bohm) and interpenetrate all energy and substance in the explicate order. Still said that Mind gives meaning to and directs the Motion of Matter, each planet, blood corpuscle, and atom.

4. **Life is a substance**, according to Still. David Bohm indicated that consciousness is a substance that exists in the implicate order to create meaning and form in the explicate order. According to William Tiller, fine substances such as consciousness, thought, and emotion exist in what he called reciprocal (wave) space. They represent the spiritual aspect of reality, something that can be measured in wave space as readily as matter is measured in particulate space with Tiller's new mathematical model.

5. **Morphogenetic fields** (Sheldrake) generate within the implicate order as expressions of consciousness. They are templates for structures in the explicate order. The attractors of chaos theory have similar attributes. Still referred to these patterns of energy as the plans and specifications. The author also chooses to think of individuations of spirit, or souls, the energetic essence of beings, as expressions of morphogenetic fields.

6. **Material substance**, which Still called Matter, develops as atoms emerge from the implicate order and appear in the explicate order (Bohm) or Terrestrial realm (Still). Bohm said that ephemeral subatomic particles appear from and disappear into the implicate order through holomovement. In creating individuated entities, morphogenetic fields in the implicate order direct the coalescence of atoms in the explicate order.

7. **Entities of matter** individuate, manifesting as galaxies, star systems, planets, minerals, air, water, plants, and animals, based on the laws of physics. Still indicated that the realms of the Celestial and Terrestrial reciprocate; that is, Mind and spirit reciprocate with Matter to form worlds and beings. The implicate order includes the explicate order.

8. **Motion** (Still) is the visible effect of the vivifying spark, the life force. Existing in the implicate order, life itself cannot be described as having motion, but it serves as the impetus for motion of substance in the explicate order. Motion includes thermodynamics, chemistry, physiology, biomechanics, and all detectable movement in the Terrestrial.

9. **Motion manifests life.** In the physical realm, a sleeping person looks the same as a recently deceased person, except for motion. Vital signs are all expressions of motion. In the physical realm, "We know life only by the motion of material bodies."[1]

10. **Biogen** (Still) is the most basic living matter, in which the Life Force expresses definite arrangements by which it unites with and moves matter. Biogen results from united action in which the Terrestrial and Celestial reciprocate to create living tissue (protoplasm) that manifests motion and growth. "Life terrestrial has motion and power; the celestial bodies have knowledge and wisdom. . . . The result is faultless perfection, because the earth-life shows in material forms the wisdom of the God of the celestial" (Still 1892, 251).

11. **The Terrestrial reciprocates with the Celestial** for the benefit of both; structure (Terrestrial) receives the benefit of life-giving resonance, and function (Celestial) receives the benefit of a vehicle in which it can reside.

12. Once **structure** (the material component) is established, the energy of the unseen **function** (the spiritual component) depends on the original orderly form that spirit created for its ongoing resonant residence. The ongoing union between life and matter depends on free and absolute motion.

13. If the **distortion of the structure** of a living organism

occurs from trauma or other influence and if the distortion exceeds the power of the function to restore it to the form that function originally created, then function (spirit) requires assistance from outside to restore the original structure. The original function was sufficiently powerful to create the original structure in the embryo, which is mostly fluid. However, in the adult, because structure has co-opted fluid, the power of function alone may not be sufficient to recreate the original structure if the distortion is too severe.

14. **Function** (the spiritual quality) within the structure of the living organism **suffers from distortion** of structure (the material quality). In such rigid structural distortions, it becomes more difficult to maintain reciprocity between structure and function.

15. **Disease** and death result from the dissonance between the perfection of the immaterial and the distortion of the material.

16. **Intervention** to restore originality of structure or to energize function, both of which can restore original resonance, also affords the system that which we call health and life.

17. A **vital resonance** demonstrates the harmony of spirit and form, the epitome of health. Conversely, a lack of resonance reveals a form struggling to fully live, leading to disease and dysfunction.

18. **Health** is the natural result of spirit's investment in the physical body. Spirit's vitality enlivens all aspects of the living organism: anatomy, physiology, biochemistry, emotion, thought, and behavior.

19. The perfection of the original form and function come from the Celestial, or divinity. Therefore, **healing is a divine act**.

20. **Fluids** deliver Health. These fluids surround and exist within cells, as well as within blood and lymphatic vessels.

21. The **brain** is the battery and powers the system through nerves. It derives its charge from its dynamo-like activity. It also charges the cerebrospinal fluid that surrounds it and the interstitial fluid of the rest of the organism.

22. The **integration** of the whole organism occurs by the action of the nervous system together with endocrine and immune functions. These functions all impinge on the extracellular matrix.

23. The **connective tissues**, including the extracellular matrix and cytoskeleton, act to integrate the whole, behaving as primitive nervous, endocrine, and immune systems.

24. **All organs** and systems of the organism serve each other through the integrating systems: nervous, endocrine, immune, and connective tissues. The connective tissues not only integrate but also contain the organism, its activity, and its behavior, which are charged by spirit.

25. **Health** depends on the mutual functioning of all these systems.

NOTES

Introduction

1   Harvey W (1957). 'De Motu Cordis' (Movement of the heart and blood in animals). Translated from Latin. Oxford: Blackwell.

2   Sutherland W (1939). *The Cranial Bowl*. Mankato, MN: Free Press.

Chapter One

1   In Booth ER (1905). *History of Osteopathy*. Cincinnati, OH: Press of Jennings and Graham, 63. [Work hereafter cited in text.]

2   *Glossary of Osteopathic Terminology* (1999). Prepared and revised by the Glossary Review Committee, Educational Council on Osteopathic Principles, American Association of Colleges of Osteopathic Medicine. In D'Alonzo G (ed.)(2000). *AOA Yearbook and Directory of Osteopathic Physicians*. Chicago: American Osteopathis Association, 863.

3   Still, AT (1892). *The Philosophy and Mechanical Principles of Osteopathy*. Republished 1986. Kirksville, MO: Osteopathic Enterprise, 319. [Work hereafter cited in text.]

4   Still, AT (1899). *The Philosophy of Osteopathy*. Fifth reprint, 1977. Indianapolis, IN: American Academy of Osteopathy, 268.

5   Still, AT (1908). *Autobiography of Andrew T Still*. Reprinted 1981. Indianapolis, IN: American Academy of Osteopathy, 402. [Work hereafter cited in text.]

6   Still, AT (1910). *Osteopathy: Research and Practice*. Reprinted 1992. Seattle, WA: Eastland Press, 293.

7   Hazzard C (1900). *The Practice and Applied Therapeutics of Osteopathy*. Kirksville, MO: Chas Hazzard, 266.

8   Hulett GD (1903). *A Text Book of the Principles of Osteopathy*. Kirksville, MO: Journal Printing Co., 366.

9   Booth, *History of Osteopathy*, 428.

10 Lane MA (1918). *Dr. Andrew Taylor Still, Founder of Osteopathy*. Chicago: The Osteopathic Publishing Co., 217.

11 McConnell CP and Teall CC (1920). *The Practice of Osteopathy*. Fourth Ed. Kirksville, MO: Journal Printing Co., 808.

12 Castlio Y, ed. (1935). *Collected Papers of Dr. George J. Conley*. Kansas City, MO: Kansas City College of Osteopathy and Surgery, 432.

13   Hildreth AG (1938). *The Lengthening Shadow of Dr. Andrew Taylor Still*. Kirksville, MO: Journal Printing Co., 464. [Work hereafter cited in text.]

14   Proposed tenets of osteopathic medicine and principles for patient care (2002). *JAOA*, 102(2):63–65.

15   Weaver C (1938). The three primary brain vesicles and the three cranial vertebrae. *JAOA,* 37:348.

16   Sutherland WG, in Truhlar, RE (1950). *Doctor A. T. Still in the Living*. Self-published, 9.

17   Booth, *History of Osteopathy*, 428.

18   Still, *Autobiography*.

19   Still CE, Jr. (1991). *Frontier Doctor—Medical Pioneer: The Life and Times of A. T. Still and His Family*. Kirksville, MO: Thomas Jefferson University Press, 288.

20   Trowbridge C (1991). *Andrew Taylor Still: 1828–1917*. Kirksville, MO: Thomas Jefferson University Press, 234. [Work hereafter cited in text.]

21   Seffinger MA (1997). Osteopathic philosophy. In Ward RC (ed.) *Foundations for Osteopathic Medicine*. Baltimore, MD: Williams & Wilkins, 4.

22   *Glossary of Osteopathic Terminology* (1999). Prepared and revised by the Glossary Review Committee, Educational Council on Osteopathic Principles, American Association of Colleges of Osteopathic Medicine. In D'Alonzo G (ed.)(2000). *AOA Yearbook and Directory of Osteopathic Physicians*. Chicago: American Osteopathis Association, 869.

23   Patterson MM and Wurster RD (1997). Neurophysiologic system: Integration and disintegration. In Ward RC (ed.) *Foundations for Osteopathic Medicine*. Baltimore, MD: Williams & Wilkins, 137–151.

24   Patterson MM and Howell JN, eds. (1992). *The Central Connection: Somatovisceral/Viscerosomatic Interaction*. Proceedings of the 1989 American Academy of Osteopathy International Symposium. Indianapolis, IN: American Academy of Osteopathy, 298.

25   Willard FH and Patterson MM, eds. (1994). *Nociception and the Neuroendocrine-Immune Connection*. Proceedings of the 1992 American Academy of Osteopathy International Symposium. Indianapolis, IN: American Academy of Osteopathy, 327.

26   For substantial scientific literature in support of these clinical phenomena, see Patterson and Howell, *Central Connection*; Willard and Patternson, *Nociception and the Neuroendocrine-Immune Connection.*

27   Jones LH (1995). *Jones Strain-CounterStrain*. Boise, ID: Jones Strain-CounterStrain, Inc., 163.

28   For a full review of osteopathic techniques, see Ward RC, ed. (2003). *Foundations for Osteopathic Medicine*. Second Ed. Baltimore, MD: Lippincott Williams & Wilkins, 819–1153.

29   *Glossary of Osteopathic Terminology* (1999). Prepared and revised by the Glossary Review Committee, Educational Council on Osteopathic Principles, American Association of Colleges of Osteopathic Medicine. In D'Alonzo G

(ed.)(2000). *AOA Yearbook and Directory of Osteopathic Physicians.* Chicago: American Osteopathis Association, 869.

30   Still AT (1895). Progress of osteopathy. *J Osteop*, 1:3.

31   Still AT (1896). Osteopathic notes. *J Osteop*, 2:3.

32   Goddeau RP (2002). Wrestling with the meaning of osteopathic medicine. *DO*, 43(3):15–17.

33   Still, *Frontier Doctor,* 288.

34   Hulett, *Text Book,* 16.

35   Kinne-Saffran E and Kinne RKH (1999). Vitalism and synthesis of urea. *Am J Nephrol*, 19:290–294.

36   Rey R (1995). Vitalism, disease and society. *Clio Med*, 29:274.

37   Truhlar, *Doctor A. T. Still*, Preface.

38   In Webster G (1917). *Concerning Osteopathy.* Plimpton Press, 2.

39   Paulus S (2001). Health and the therapeutic process. *Inter Linea: J Osteop Philos*, 3(3):6.

40   A. T. Still, in Schnucker R, ed. (1991). *Early Osteopathy in the Words of A. T. Still.* Kirksville, MO: Thomas Jefferson University Press, 172.

Chapter Two

1   Ellis A, Wiseman N, and Boss K (1989). *Grasping the Wind.* Brookline, MA: Paradigm Publications.

2   Hazzard C (1900). *The Practice and Applied Therapeutics of Osteopathy.* Kirksville, MO: Chas Hazzard.

3   Hulett GD (1903). *A Text Book of the Principles of Osteopathy.* Kirksville, MO: Journal Printing Co. [Work hereafter cited in text.]

4   Booth ER (1905). *History of Osteopathy.* Cincinnati, OH: Press of Jennings and Graham. [Work hereafter cited in text.]

5   Lane MA (1918). *Dr. Andrew Taylor Still, Founder of Osteopathy.* Chicago: The Osteopathic Publishing Co.

6   McConnell CP and Teall CC (1920). *The Practice of Osteopathy.* Fourth Ed. Kirksville, MO: Journal Printing Co.

7   Hildreth AG (1938). *The Lengthening Shadow of Dr. Andrew Taylor Still.* Kirksville MO: Journal Printing Co. [Work hereafter cited in text.]

8   Still AT (1892). *The Philosophy and Mechanical Principles of Osteopathy.* Republished 1986. Kirksville, MO: Osteopathic Enterprise, 27. [Work hereafter cited in text.]

9   Wilber K, ed. (1982). *The Holographic Paradigm and Other Paradoxes.* Boulder, CO and London: Shambhala, 301.

10   Still AT (1908). *Autobiography of Andrew T Still.* Reprinted 1981. Indianapolis, IN: American Academy of Osteopathy, 94. [Work hereafter cited in text.]

11   Holmes O (1892). *Medical Essays, 1842–1882.* Boston: Houghton Mifflin, 203.

12   Pischinger A (1991). *Matrix and Matrix Regulation: Basis for a Holistic Theory*

of Medicine. Heine, H (ed.). Brussels, Belgium: Haug International, 221. [Work hereafter cited in text.]

13   Trowbridge C (1991). *Andrew Taylor Still: 1828–1917*. Kirksville, MO: Thomas Jefferson University Press, 107–109. [Work hereafter cited in text.]

14   Swedenborg E (1882). *The Brain, Vol. 1: The Cerebrum and Its Parts*. Tafel RL (ed. & tr.). London: James Speirs, Swedenborg Library Academy of the New Church, 794. [Work hereafter cited in text.]

15   Swedenborg E (1887). *The Brain, Vol. 2: The Pituitary Gland, the Cerebellum, and the Medulla Oblongata*. Tafel RL (ed. & tr.). London: James Speirs, Swedenborg Library Academy of the New Church, 645.

16   Swedenborg E (1938). *The Cerebrum, Vol. 1*. Acton A (ed.). Philadelphia: Swedenborg Scientific Association, 731.

17   Swedenborg E (1938). *The Cerebrum: Anatomical Plates*. Acton A (ed.). Philadelphia: Swedenborg Scientific Association, n.p.

18   Swedenborg E (1769). *Intercourse of the Soul and the Body*. Republished 1947. London: The Swedenborg Society, 61. [Work hereafter cited in text.]

19   Lee RP (2000). Spirituality in osteopathic medicine. *AAO J*, (Winter): 31–36. [Work hereafter cited in text.]

20   Helms JM (1995). *Acupuncture Energetics: A Clinical Approach for Physicians*. Berkeley, CA: Medical Acupuncture Publishers, 759.

21   Kaptchuck TJ (1983). *The Web That Has No Weaver*. New York: Congdon & Weed, 402.

22   Reported in the Topeka, KS, *Daily Capitol*, December 8, 1907.

23   Rael J (2002). *In the House of Shattering Light: The Life and Teachings of a Native American Mystic*. Self-published, 37. [Work hereafter cited in text.]

24   Alvord LA (1999). *The Scalpel and the Silver Bear*. New York: Bantam Books, 120–127. [Work hereafter cited in text.]

25   Sheldrake R (1981). *A New Science of Life*. Los Angeles: Jeremy Tarcher, 229. [Work hereafter cited in text.]

26   Capra F (1991). *The Tao of Physics*. Boston: Shambala, 366.

27   Gerber R (1988). *Vibrational Medicine*. Santa Fe, NM: Bear & Co, 558.

28   Handoll N (2000). *The Anatomy of Potency*. Portland, OR: Stillness Press, 178.

29   Mandelbrot B (1977). *The Fractal Geometry of Nature*. New York: W.H. Freeman, 5. [Work hereafter cited in text.]

30   Dossey L (1999). *Reinventing Medicine*. New York: HarperSanFrancisco. [Work hereafter cited in text.]

31   Denney M (2002). Walking the quantum talk. *IONS Noetic Sci Rev*, (June–August):19–23. [Work hereafter cited in text.]

32   Still AT (1910). *Osteopathy: Research and Practice*. Reprinted 1992. Seattle, WA: Eastland Press, par. 905.

33   Tiller W (1997). *Science and Human Transformation: Subtle Energies, Intentionality, and Consciousness*. Walnut Creek, CA: Pavior Publishing.

34   Tiller W, Dibble W, and Kohane M (2001). *Conscious Acts of Creation: The Emergence of a New Physics*. Walnut Creek, CA: Pavior Publishing.

35   Tiller W (2002). Personal communication.

36   Grimes D (2003). Universe void fuels fear of "cosmic poof." *Herald-Tribune* (Sarasota, FL), February 24:E1.

37   Shimotsu J (1982). The simplified and revised abridged edition of changing reality by Marilyn Ferguson. In Wilber K (ed.) *The Holographic Paradigm*. Boulder, CO: Shambhala, 126. [Work hereafter cited in text.]

38   Brohm D (1978). In Wilber K (ed.) *The Holographic Paradigm*. Boulder, CO: Shambhala.

39   Rause V (2001). The science of God. *Los Angeles Times Magazine,* July 15.

40   Sorli A (2001). Additional roundness of space-time and unknown vacuum energies in living organisms. *Frontier Perspect,* 10(2):6–7.

41   Emoto M (1999). *Messages from Water, Vol. 1.* Tokyo: I.H.M. General Research Institute, HADO Kyoikusha Co.

42   Emoto M (2002). *Messages from Water, Vol. 2.* Tokyo: I.H.M. General Research Institute, HADO Kyoishuka Co.

43   Schwenk T (1996). *Sensitive Chaos.* Second Ed. London: Rudolf Steiner Press, 144, illus. [Work hereafter cited in text.]

44   Blechschmidt E (1977). *The Beginnings of Human Life.* New York: Springer-Verlag, 128.

45   Jealous J (1993). Personal communication.

Chapter Three

1   Hazzard C (1900). *The Practice and Applied Therapeutics of Osteopathy.* Kirksville, MO: Chas Hazzard.

2   Lane MA (1918). *Dr. Andrew Taylor Still, Founder of Osteopathy.* Chicago: The Osteopathic Publishing Co.

3   McConnell CP and Teall CC (1920). *The Practice of Osteopathy.* Fourth Ed. Kirksville, MO: Journal Printing Co.

4   Trowbridge C (1991). *Andrew Taylor Still: 1828–1917.* Kirksville, MO: Thomas Jefferson University Press, 187. [Work hereafter cited in text.]

5   McConnell C (1913). Osteopathy in the light of evolution. *J Am Osteopath Assoc,* 12:499–505.

6   Walter G (1992). The First School of Osteopathic Medicine. Kirksville, MO: Thomas Jefferson University Press, 30.

7   Hildreth AG (1938). *The Lengthening Shadow of Dr. Andrew Taylor Still.* Kirksville, MO: Journal Printing Co.

8   Conley G (1935). *Collected Papers of George J. Conley.* Castlio Y (ed.). Kansas City: Kansas City College of Osteopathy and Surgery, 432.

9   Litton H (1944). *Handbook of Osteopathic Technique by the Staff of the Department of Osteopathic Technique.* Los Angeles: College of Physicians and Surgeons, 153.

10   Hulett GD (1903). *A Text Book of the Principles of Osteopathy.* Kirksville, MO: Journal Printing Co.

11   Booth ER (1905). *History of Osteopathy.* Cincinnati, OH: Press of Jennings

and Graham. [Work hereafter cited in text.]

12   Sutherland W (1939). *The Cranial Bowl*. Mankato, MN: Self-published. Republished 1986, Indianapolis, IN: Cranial Academy.

13   Lippincott H (1949). The osteopathic technique of Wm G Sutherland, DO. *AAO Yearbook*, 1–24.

14   Sutherland A (1962). *With Thinking Fingers*. Indianapolis, IN: Cranial Academy, 13. [Work hereafter cited in text.]

15   Magoun H (1951). *Osteopathy in the Cranial Field*. Republished 1997. Indianapolis, IN: Sutherland Cranial Teaching Foundation. [Work hereafter cited in text.]

16   Magoun H (1976). *Osteopathy in the Cranial Field*. Third Ed. Indianapolis, IN: Cranial Academy.

17   Kahn F (1943). *Man in Structure and Function, Vol. 1*. New York: Alfred A. Knopf, 103.

18   Todd TW and Lyon DW, Jr. (1924). Endocranial suture closure, its progress and age relationship, I. Adult males of white stock. *Am J Phys Anthrop*, 7:325–384.

19   Todd TW and Lyon DW, Jr. (1925). Endocranial suture closure, its progress and age relationship, II. Ectocranial suture closure in adult males of white stock. *Am J Phys Anthrop*, 8:23–45.

20   Todd TW and Lyon DW, Jr. (1925). Endocranial suture closure, its progress and age relationship, III. Endocranial closure in adult males of Negro stock. *Am J Phys Anthrop*, 8:47–71.

21   Todd TW and Lyon DW, Jr. (1925). Endocranial suture closure, its progress and age relationship, IV. Ectocranial closure in adult males of Negro stock. *Am J Phys Anthrop*, 8:149–168.

22   Ashley-Montagu M (1938). Aging of the skull. *Am J Phys Anthrop*, 23:355–375.

23   Singer R (1953). Estimation of age from cranial suture closure: Report on its unreliability. *J Forensic Med*, 1:52–59.

24   Hershkovitz I et al. (1997). Why do we fail in aging the skull from the sagittal suture? *Am J Phys Anthrop*, 103:393–399.

25   King H (1999). Articular mobility of the cranial bones: A review of the research and status of the support for further research on osteopathy in the cranial field. *Cranial Lett*, 52(4):11–13.

26   Pritchard J et al. (1956). The structure and development of cranial and facial sutures. *J Anat* (London), 90:73–86.

27   Moss M (1957). Experimental alteration of sutural area morphology. *Anat Rec*, 127:569–589.

28   Moss M (1958). Fusion of the frontal suture in the rat. *Am J Anat*, 102:141–165.

29   Moss M (1960). Inhibition and stimulation of sutural fusion in the rat calvaria. *Anat Rec*, 136: 457–467.

30   Moss M (1959). The pathogenesis of premature cranial synostosis in man.

Acta Anat, 37:351–370.

31 Frymann V (1971). A study of the rhythmic motions of the living cranium. *J Am Osteop Assoc,* 70:1–18.

32 Hubbard R et al. (1971). Flexure of cranial sutures. *J Biomechanics,* 4:491–496.

33 Hubbard R (1971). Flexure of layered cranial bone. *J Biomechanics,* 4:251–263.

34 St. Pierre et al. (1976). The detection of relative movements of cranial bones. *J Am Osteopath Assoc,* 76:289.

35 Retzlaff E et al. (1979). Aging of cranial sutures in humans [Abstract]. *Anat Rec,* 193:663.

36 Retzlaff E et al. (1979). Age related changes in human cranial sutures. In *Proceedings of the 23rd Annual American Osteopathy Association Research Convention.* 14.

37 Retzlaff E et al. (1978). Cranial suture morphology. In *Proceedings of the 2nd World Congress on Pain, International Association for the Study of Pain, Vol. 1.* 68.

38 Retzlaff E et al. (1985). The role of the cranial ligaments in primates. *Anat Rec,* 211:159–160.

39 Kokich V et al. (1979). Craniofacial sutures. In *Aging in Nonhuman Primates.* New York: Van Nostrand Reinhold, 356–368.

40 Retzlaff E et al. (1978). Aging of cranial sutures in Macaca nemestrina. *Anat Rec,* 190:52.

41 Retzlaff E et al. (1976). The structures of cranial bone sutures. *J Am Osteopath Assoc,* 75:106–107.

42 Michael D & Retzlaff E (1975). A preliminary study of cranial bone movement in the squirrel monkey. *J Am Osteopath Assoc,* 74:866–869.

43 Kokich V (1976). Age changes in the human frontozygomatic suture from 20 to 95 years. *Am J Orthodont,* 69:411–430.

44 Adams T et al. (1992). Parietal bone mobility in the anesthetized cat. *J Am Osteopath Assoc,* 92(5):599–622.

45 Moskalenko Y et al. (1996). Bioengineering support of the cranial osteopathic treatment. *Med Biol Eng Comput,* 34 (suppl 1, part 2):185–186.

46 Moskalenko Y et al. (1998). Applications of bio-impedance for the study of hemo and CSF dynamics in the human head. In Riu P et al.(ed.)*Proceedings of the Xth International Conference on Electrical and Bio-Impedance.* Barcelona, Spain, 91–94.

47 Moskalenko Y (1998). The phenomenology and mechanisms of cranial bone fluctuations. In *Proceedings of 1st Russian Symposium.*

48 Heisey S and Adams T (1993). Role of cranial bone mobility in cranial compliance. *Neurosurgery,* 33(5):869–876.

49 Moskalenko Y et al. (1999). Periodic mobility of cranial bones in humans. *Hum Physiol,* 25(1):51–58.

50 Upledger J and Vredevoogd J. ( ). *Craniosacral Therapy Slide Series.* Palm Beach

Gardens, FL: The Upledger Institute.

51 Sutherland W (1998). *Contributions of Thought*. Second Ed. Fort Worth, TX: Sutherland Cranial Teaching Foundation.

52 Lee R (2000). Tensegrity. *Cranial Lett*, 53(3):10–13.

53 Pienta K and Coffey D (1991). Cellular harmonic information transfer through a tissue tensegrity-matrix system. *Med Hypothesis,* 34:88–95. Quotation on p.91, italics added.

54 Levin S (1997). A different approach to the mechanics of the human pelvis: tensegrity. In Vleeming A et al. (eds.) *Movement, Stability, and Low Back Pain: The Essential Role of the Pelvis.* New York: Churchill Livingstone.

55 Wales A (1999). *Basic Course Manual.* Indianapolis, IN: Cranial Academy.

56 Retzlaff E et al. (1975). Cranial bone mobility. *J Am Osteopath Assoc*, 74:138–146.

57 Still, AT (1908). *Autobiography of Andrew T Still*. Reprinted 1981. Indianapolis, IN: American Academy of Osteopathy, 302. [Work hereafter cited in text.]

58 Davies P (1992). *The Mind of God: The Scientific Basis for a Rational World.* New York: Simon & Schuster, 227.

59 Hawkins D (1995). *Power vs. Force: The Hidden Determinants of Human Behavior.* Carlsbad, CA: Hay House, 43.

60 Sutherland W (1990). *Teachings in the Science of Osteopathy*. Wales A (ed.). Fort Worth, TX: Sutherland Cranial Teaching Foundation, 51–64. [Work hereafter cited in text.]

61 Still AT (1897). *Autobiography of A. T. Still.* Self-published, 182.

61a Lecain, Alliot, Laine, Calas, and Pessac. Alpha isoform of smooth muscle actin is expressed in astrocytes in vitro and in vivo. *J Neurosci Res* 28(4):601-6, 1991.

62 Weaver C (1936). The cranial vertebrae. *J Am Osteop Assoc,* 37(3):328–336.

63 Weaver C (1936). The cranial vertebrae, II. *J Am Osteop Assoc*, 37(4):374–379.

64 Weaver C (1936). The cranial vertebrae, III. *J Am Osteop Assoc*, 37(5):421–424.

65 Weaver C (1936). Etiologic importance of the cranial intervertebral articulations. *J Am Osteop Assoc*, 37(7):515–525.

66 Jenkins CO et al. (1971). Modulation resembling Traube-Hering waves recorded in the human brain. *Europ Neurol*, 5:1–6.

67 Greitz D et al. (1992). Pulsatile brain movement and associated hydrodynamics studied by magnetic resonance phase imaging: The Monro-Kellie doctrine revisited. *Diagn Neuroradiol*, 34:370–380.

68 Wales A (1986). Personal communication.

69 Still AT (1899). *The Philosophy of Osteopathy*. Fifth reprint, 1977. Indianapolis, IN: American Academy of Osteopathy, 38–39.

70 Jealous J (2002). Sutherland memorial lecture. *Cranial Lett*, 55(3):3.

71 Truhlar R (1950). *Doctor A. T. Still in the Living*. Self-published, 154.

72 Paulus S (2001). Health and the therapeutic process. *Inter Linea, J Osteop Philos*, 3(3):8.

73 Lee RP (2002). Fluids: Matter in motion. *Cranial Lett*. Part 1: 55(4):4–11, Part 2: 56(1):7–10.

74 Paulus, Health and the therapeutic process, 9.

75 Bohm D (1985). *Brain/Mind Bull*, 10:10.

76 Lovelock J (1979). *Gaia: A New Look at Life on Earth*. Oxford: Oxford University Press.

77 Goldberger A, Bhargava V, and West B (1985). Nonlinear dynamics of the heartbeat. *Physica D,* 17.

78 Mackay M and Glass L (1977). Oscillation and chaos in physiological control systems. *Science,* 197.

79 Lewis M and Rees D (1985). Fractal surfaces of proteins. *Science,* 230.

Chapter Four

1   Kimberly P (1985). Scott memorial lecture. Kirksville College of Osteopathic Medicine, Kirksville, MO.

2   Good W (1981). Water relations of altered body functions. *Med Hypothesis*, 7:85–110.

3   Lee RP (2002). Fluids: Matter in motion. *Cranial Lett*, 55(4):6–11.

4   Saenger W (1987). Structure and dynamics of water surrounding biomolecules. *Ann Rev Biophys*, 16:93–114.

5   Urry D (1995). Elastic biomolecular machines. *Sci Am,*January: 64–69.

6   Schwenk T (1996). *Sensitive Chaos*. Second Ed. London: Rudolf Steiner Press, 73. [Work hereafter cited in text.]

7   Cowin S et al. (1991). Candidates for the mechanosensory system in bone. *J Biochem Eng*, 113:191–197.

8   Becker R (1990). *Cross Currents*. Los Angeles: Jeremy Tarcher, 147.

9   Nordenström B (1983). *Biologically Closed Electric Circuits*. Stockholm: Nordic Medical Publications.

10 Becker, *Cross Currents*. [Work hereafter cited in text.]

11 Becker R (1988). *The Body Electric*. Los Angeles: Jeremy Tarcher.

12 Blechschmidt E (1977). *The Beginnings of Human Life*. New York: Springer-Verlag, 223.

13 Lee RP (2003). Fluids: Matter in motion, II. *Cranial Lett*, 56(1):7–10, illus.

14 Emoto M (1999). *Messages from Water, Vol. 1*. Tokyo: I.H.M. General Research Institute, HADO Kyoikusha Co.

15 Emoto M (2002). *Messages from Water, Vol. 2*. Tokyo: I.H.M. General Research Institute, HADO Kyoishuka Co.

16 Berridge MJ and Rapp PE (1979). A comparative survey of the function, mechanism and control of cellular oscillators. *J Exp Biol*, 81:217–279.

17 Rapp PE (1979). An atlas of cellular oscillators. *J Exp Biol*, 81:281–306.

18 Klevecs RR et al. (1984). Cellular clocks and oscillators. *Int Rev Cytol*, 86:97–128.

19 Barral JP (1989). *Visceral Manipulation*. Seattle, WA: Eastland Press.

20 Cohen D (1968). Magnetoencephalography: Evidence of magnetic fields produced by alpha-rhythm currents. *Science,* 161:784–786.

21 Feinberg D (1992). Modern concepts of brain motion and cerebrospinal fluid

flow. *Radiology*, 185:630–632.

22   duBoulay G (1966). Pulsatile movements in the CSF pathways. *Br J Radiol*, 39:255–262.

23   Bergstrand G et al. (1985). Cardiac gated MR imaging of cerebrospinal fluid flow. *J Comput Assist Tomogr*, 9:1003–1006.

24   Feinberg D and Mark A (1986). Cerebrospinal fluid flow evaluated by inner volume magnetic resonance velocity imaging. *Acta Radiol Suppl* (Stockholm), 369:766.

25   Feinberg D and Mark A (1987). Human brain motion and cerebrospinal fluid circulation demonstrated with MR velocity imaging. *Radiology*, 163:793–799.

26   Enzmann D and Pelc N (1992). Brain motion: Measurement with phase-contrast MR imaging. *Radiology*, 185:653–660.

27   Poncelet et al. (1992). Brain parenchyma motion: Measurement with cine echo-planar MR imaging. *Radiology*, 185:645–651.

28   Goldbeter A (1996). *Biochemical Oscillations and Cellular Rhythms: The Molecular Bases of Periodic and Chaotic Behavi*or. Cambridge, UK: Cambridge University Press, 344–347.

29   Moskalenko Y and Frymann V et al. (2003). Physiological background of the cranial rhythmic impulse and the primary respiratory mechanism. *AAOJ*, 13(2):21–33.

30   Nelson K, Sergueef N, and Glonek T (2003). Wave phenomena: The Traube-Hering oscillation and the cranial rhythmic impulse. Lecture given at the PRM Research Symposium/SCTF Continuing Studies Program, Bloomingdale, IL.

31   Moskalenko Y and Frymann V (2003). Wave phenomena; circulatory dynamics. Lecture given at the PRM Research Symposium/SCTF Continuing Studies Program, Bloomingdale, IL.

32   Traube L (1865). Ueber periodische Thatigkeits-Aeusserungen des vasomotorischen und Hemmungs-Nervenzentrums. *Cbl Med Wiss*, 56:881–885.

33   Hering E (1869). Über Athembewegungen des Gefäßsystems. *Sitz Ber Akad Wiss Wien Mathe-Naturwiss Kl Anat*, 60:829–856.

34   Mayer S (1869). Uber spontane Blutdruckschwankugen. *Sitz Ber Akad Wiss Wien Mathe-Nuturwiss Kl Anat*, 60:829–856.

35   Lundberg N (1960). Continuous recording and control of ventricular fluid pressure in neurosurgical practice. *Acta Psychiat Neurol Scand*, 36:suppl 149.

36   Jenkins CO, Campbell JK, and White DN (1971). Modulation resembling Traube-Hering waves recorded in the human brain. *Europ Neurol*, 5:1–6.

37   Vern B et al. (1988). Low-frequency oscillations of cortical oxidative metabolism in waking and sleep. *J Cereb Blood Flow Metab*, 8:215–226.

38   Vern B et al. (1997). Interhemispheric synchrony of slow oscillations of cortical blood volume and cytochrome aa3 redox state in unanesthetized rabbits. *Brain Res*, 775:233–239.

39   Dora E and Kovach A (1981). Metabolic and vascular volume oscillations in the

cat brain cortex. *Acta Physiol Acad Sci Hung*, 53:261–275.

40 Mayevsky A and Ziv I (1991). Oscillations of cortical oxidative metabolism and microcirculation in the ischemic brain. *Neurol Res*, 13:39–47.

41 Clark L, Misrahy G, and Fox R (1958). Chronically implanted polygraphic electrodes. *J Appl Physiol*, 13:85–91

42 Cooper R et al. (1966). Regional control of cerebral vascular reactivity and oxygen supply in man. *Brain Res*, 3:174–191.

43 Gretchin V and Borovikova V (1982). *Slow Non-electrical Processes in the Evaluation of the Functional State of the Brain in Man.* Leningrad: Nauka, 172.

44 Kilibaeva G, Demchenko I, and Moskalenko Y (1988). Structural-functional module of the rat brain cortical microcirculatory network. *Sechenov Physiol J*, 74(9):1235–1242.

45 Moskalenko Y (1980). *Biophysical Aspects of Cerebral Circulation*. New York: Pergamon Press, 111–147.

46 Hudetz A, Roman R, and Harder D (1992). Spontaneous flow oscillations in the cerbral cortex during acute changes in mean arterial pressure. *J Cereb Blood Flow Metab*, 12:491–499.

47 Vern B et al. (1997). Correlation of increases in cortical blood volume and cytochrome aa3 oxidation with enhanced γ-electrocorticographic activity and eye movement bursts during REM sleep in cats. *Ann Neurol*, 42:458.

48 Biswal B et al. (1995). Functional connectivity in the motor cortex of resting human brain using echo-planar MRI. *MRM*, 34:537–541.

49 Biswal B et al. (1997). Hypercapnia reversibly suppresses low-frequency fluctuations in the human motor cortex during rest using echo-planar MRI. *J Cereb Blood Flow Metab*, 17:301–308.

50 Frymann V (1971). A study of the rhythmic motions of the living cranium. *J Amer Osteopath Assoc*, 70:928–945.

51 Moskalenko Y et al. (1999). Periodic mobility of cranial bones in humans. *Hum Physiol*, 25(1):51–58.

52 Moskalenko Y and Frymann V et al. (2001). Slow rhythmic oscillations within the human cranium: Phenomenology, origin, and informational significance. *Hum Physiol*, 27(2):171–178.

53 Moskalenko and Frymann, Wave phenomena; circulatory dynamics.

54 Nelson KE, Sergueef NS, Lipinski CM, Chapman AR, and Glonek T (2001). The cranial rhythmic impulse related to the Traube-Hering-Mayer oscillation: Comparing laser-Doppler flowmetry and palpation. *J Am Osteop Assoc*, 101(3):163–173.

55 Sergueef N, Nelson KE, and Glonek T (2002). The effect of cranial manipulation upon the Traube Hering Meyer oscillation. *Alter Ther Health Med*, 8(6):74–76.

56 Sergueef N, Nelson KE, and Glonek T (in review). Cranial manipulation induces sequential changes in blood flow velocity on demand. *Am Acad Osteop J*, 14(3):15–17.

57 Verbal reports of several clinicians who offered spontaneous accounts of cases

that they had personally attended, corroborating one another's findings that the PRM persists, sometimes for extended periods of time after the standard signs of life have ceased. PRM ResearchSymposium/SCTF Continuing Studies Program, Bloomingdale, IL, Oct. 2003.

58 Pischinger A (1991). *Matrix and Matrix Regulation: Basis for a Holistic Theory of Medicine.* Heine, H (ed.). Brussels, Belgium: Haug International, 221. [Work hereafter cited in text.]

60 Nordenstrom, *Biologically Closed Electric Circuits.*

61 Shamos M and Lavine L (1967). Piezoelectricity as a fundamental property of biological tissues. *Nature,* 1967(Jan. 21):267–269.

62 Still, AT (1908). *Autobiography of Andrew T Still.* Reprinted 1981. Indianapolis, IN: American Academy of Osteopathy, 402. [Work hereafter cited in text.]

63 Oschman J (2000). *Energy Medicine.* Edinburgh, UK: Churchill Livingstone, 275.

64 Mitchell P (1976). Vectorial chemistry and the molecular mechanics of chemiosmotic coupling: power transmission by proticity. *Biochem Soc Trans,* 4:399–430.

65 Deshmukh V (1991). Cascading morphoregulatory energy and the biological form: Theory and reality. *Med Hypothesis,* 35:59–67. [Work hereafter cited in text.]

66 Fulford R. (1988). *Energy and Osteopathy: A CME Course.* Indianapolis, IN: Cranial Academy.

67 Fulford R (2003). *Are We on the Path? The Collected Works of Robert Fulford, DO, FCA.* Cisler T (ed.). Indianapolis, IN: Cranial Academy, 95.

68 Comeaux Z (2002). *Robert Fulford, D.O. and the Philosopher Physician.* Seattle, WA: Eastland Press.

69 Viidik A (1996). Tendons and ligaments. In Comper W (ed.). *Extracellular Matrix, Vol. 1: Tissue Function.* Amsterdam: Harwood Academic Publishers, 304.

70 Hay E (1981). Extracellular matrix. *J Cell Biol,* 91(3):205s–223s.

71 Marlowe R et al. (1999). Mediation of a phase transition in hyaluronate films by the counterions Li, Cs, Mg, and Ca as observed by infrared spectroscopy, optical microscopy, and optical birefringence. *J Biomol Struct Dyn,* 17(3):607–616.

72 Vercruysse K, Ziebell M, and Prestwich G (1999). Control of enzymatic degradation of hyaluronan by divalent cations. *Carbohydr Res,* 318:26–37.

73 Rubin K et al. (1996). Molecular recognition of the extracellular matrix by cell surface receptors. In Comper W (ed.) *Extracellular Matrix, Vol. 2: Molecular Components and Interactions.* Amsterdam: Harwood Academic Publishers, 278. [Work hereafter cited in text.]

74 Peterson B, ed. (1979). *The Collected Papers of Irvin M. Korr.* Indianapolis, IN: American Academy of Osteopathy.

75 King H, ed. (1997). *The Collected Papers of Irvin M. Korr, Vol. 2.* Indianapolis,

IN: American Academy of Osteopathy.

76 Jaffe L (1999). Organization of early development by calcium patterns. *Bioessays,* 21:657–667. [Work hereafter cited in text.]

77 Ingber D (1998). The architecture of life. *Sci Am*, 1998(Jan.):48–57. [Work hereafter cited in text.]

78 Blechschmidt E (2004). *The Ontogenetic Basis of Human Anatomy*. Berkeley, CA: North Atlantic Books, 61–69.

79 Grodzinsky A et al. (1996). The role of specific macromolecules in cell-matrix interactions and in matrix function: Phsicochemical and mechanical mediators of chondrocyte biosynthesis. In Comper W (ed.) *Extracellular Matrix, Vol. 2: Molecular Components and Interactions*. Amsterdam: Harwood Academic Publishers, 310. [Work hereafter cited in text.]

80 Prajapati R et al. (2000). Mechanical loading regulates protease production by fibroblasts in three-dimensional collagen substrates. *Wound Rep Reg*, 8:226–237.

81 Pollack G (2001). *Cells, Gels and the Engines of Life*. Seattle, WA: Ebner and Sons.

82 Fröhlich H (1968). Bose condensation of strongly excited longitudinal electric modes. *Phys Lett*, 26A:402–403.

83 Fröhlich H (1988). *Biological Coherence and Response to External Stimuli*. Berlin: Springer Verlag.

84 Goldbeter, *Biochemical Oscillations and Cellular Rhythms,* 605.

85 Hess B (2000). Periodic patterns in biology. *Naturwissenschaften,* 87:199–211. [Work hereafter cited in text.]

86 Berridge MJ and Rapp PE (1979). A comparative survey of the function, mechanism and control of cellular oscillators. *J Exp Biol*, 81:221–224.

87 Gorbunova Y and Spitzer N (2002). Dynamic interactions of cyclic AMP transients and spontaneous Ca^{2+} spikes. *Nature,* 418:93–96.

88 Lee RP (2001). The primary respiratory mechanism beyond the craniospinal axis. *AAOJ*, 11(1):24–34.

89 Jealous J (1998). Personal communication.

90 Sergueef N et al. (2001). Changes in the Traube-Herring wave following cranial manipulation. *AAOJ*, 11(1):17.

91 Frymann, Study of the rhythmic motions, 928–945.

92 Upledger JE and Vredevoogd JD (1983). *Craniosacral Therapy*. Chicago: Eastland Press.

93 Geiger AJ (1992). Letter to the editor. *J Amer Osteop Assoc*, 92:1088–1093.

94 McPartland JM and Mein EA (1997). Entrainment and the cranial rhythmic impulse. *Alt Ther,* 3(1):40–45.

95 Nelson KE et al. (2001). The cranial rhythmic impulse related to the Traube-Herring-Mayer oscillation: Comparing laser-Doppler flowmetry and palpation. *J Amer Osteop Assoc*, 101(3):163–173.

96 Guyton AC and Harris JW (1951). Pressoreceptor-autonomic oscillation: A probable cause of vasomotor waves. *Am J Physiol*, 165:158.

97 Nordenström, *Biologically Closed Electric Circuits*, 358.

98 Berridge MJ and Rapp PE (1979). A comparative survey of the function, mechanism and control of cellular oscillations. *J Exp Biol*, 81:217–279.

99 Goldbeter A and Caplan SR (1976). Oscillatory enzymes. *Annu Rev Biophys Bioeng*, 5:469–476.

100 Hess B and Boiteau A (1971). Oscillatory phenomena in biochemistry. *Annu Rev Biochem*, 40:237–258.

101 Nicolis G and Prigogine I (1977). *Self-Organization in Nonequilibrium Systems*. New York: John Wiley.

102 Field RJ and Burger M (1985). *Oscillations and Traveling Waves in Chemical Systems*. New York: John Wiley.

103 Goldbeter, *Biochemical Oscillations and Cellular Rhythms*.

104 Goldbeter A, ed. (1998). Oscillations, bistability and waves in biochemical and cellular systems. *Biophys Chem*, 72:1–230.

105 Hess B (1997). Periodic patterns in biochemical reactions. *Q Rev Biophys*, 30:121–176.

106 Marhl M et al. (2000). Complex calcium oscillations and the role of mitochondria and cytosolic proteins. *Biosystems*, 57:75–86.

107 Schuster S, Marhl M, and Hofer T (2002). Modelling of simple and complex calcium oscillations: From single-cell responses to intercellular signalling. *Eur J Biochem*, 269(5):1333–1355.

108 Hertz L, Code W, and Sykova E (1992). Ions, water, and energy in brain cells: A synopsis of interrelations. *Can J Physiol Pharmacol*, 70:S100–S106.

109 Jaffe L and Créton R (1998). On the conservation of calcium wave speeds. *Cell Calcium*, 24:1–8.

110 Boudreau N and Bissell M (1996). Regulation of gene expression by the extracellular matrix. In Comper W (ed.) *Extracellular Matrix, Vol. 2: Molecular Components and Interactions*. Amsterdam: Harwood Academic Publishers, 262.

111 Goldbeter, *Biochemical Oscillations and Cellular Rhythms*.

112 Martiel J-P and Goldbeter A (1987). A model based on receptor desensitization for cyclic AMP signalling in Dictyostelium cells. *Biophys J*, 52:807–828.

113 Ingber D et al. (1994). Cellular tensegrity: Exploring how mechanical changes in the cytoskeleton regulate cell growth, migration, and tissue pattern during morphogenesis. *Int Rev Cytol*, 150:173–212.

114 Ingber D (1993). Cellular tensegrity: Defining new rules of biological design that govern the cytoskeleton. *J Cell Sci*, 104:613–627.

115 Levin S (1997). A different approach to the mechanics of the human pelvis: Tensegrity. In Vleeming A et al. (eds.) *Movement, Stability and Low Back Pain: The Essential Role of the Pelvis*. New York: Churchill Livingstone, 157–167. [Work hereafter cited in text.]

116 Lee R (2000). Tensegrity. *Cranial Lett*, 53(3):10–13.

117 Chen C and Ingber D (1999). Osteoarthritis and cartilage. *J OARSI*, 7:81–94.

118 Hill T (1981). Microfilament and microtubule assembly or disassembly against a force. *Proc Nat Acad Sci USA*, 78:5613–5617.

119 Maniotis A, Chen C, and Ingber D (1997). Demonstration of mechanical connections between integrins, cytoskeletal filaments, and nucleoplasm that stabilizes nuclear structure. *Proc Nat Acad Sci USA*, 94:849.

120 Wang N, Butler J, and Ingber D, (1993). Mechanotransduction across the cell surface and through the cytoskeleton. *Science*, 260:1124–1127. [Work hereafter cited in text.]

121 Newman S and Tomasek J (1996). Morphogenesis of connective tissues. In Comper W (ed.) *Extracellular Matrix, Vol. 2: Molecular Components and Interactions*. Amsterdam: Harwood Academic Publishers, 348.

122 Ingber D (1997). Tensegrity: The architectural basis of cellular mechanotransduction. *Annu Rev Physiol*, 59:575–599. [Work hereafter cited in text.]

123 He Y and Grinnell F (1994). Stress relaxation of fibroblasts activates a cyclic AMP signaling pathway. *J Cell Biol*, 126(2):457–464.

124 Lab M (1999). Mechanosensitivity as an integrative system in heart: An audit. *Prog Biophys Mol Biol*, 71:7–27.

125 Pienta K and Coffey D (1991). Cellular harmonic information transfer through a tissue tensegrity-matrix system. *Med Hypothesis*, 34:88–95. [Work hereafter cited in text.]

126 Ingber D and Jamieson J (1985). Cells as tensegrity structures: Architectural regulation of histodifferentiation by physical forces transduced over basement membrane. In Andersson, Gahmberg, and Kblom (eds.) *Gene Expression during Normal and Malignant Differentiation*. New York: Academic Press, 13.

127 Al-Habori M (1995). Microcompartmentation, metabolic channelling and carbohydrate metabolism. *J Biochem Cell Biol*, 27(2):123–132. [Work hereafter cited in text.]

128 Sherrinton C (1940). *'Man on His Nature', Gifford Lectures 1937/8*. Harmondsworth, UK: Penguin Books, 69–98. Quotation is on p. 247.

129 Clegg J (1992). Cellular infrastructure and metabolic organization. *Curr Topics Cell Reg*, 33:3–14.

130 Pienta K and Hoover C (1994). Coupling of cell structure to cell metabolism and function. *J Cell Biochem*, 55(1):16–21.

131 Cooper M (1995). Intercellular signaling in neuronal-glial networks. *BioSystems*, 34:65–85.

132 Stacey D and Allfrey V (1977). *J Cell Biol*, 75:807–817.

133 Wheatley D (1985). Mini-review on the possible importance of an intracellular circulation. *Life Sci*, 36:299–307. [Work hereafter cited in text.]

134 Kimelberg H and Frangakis M (1986). Volume regulation in primary astrocyte cultures. *Adv Biosci*, 61:177–186.

135 Walz W (1987). Swelling and potassium uptake in cultured astrocytes. *Can J Physiol Pharmacol*, 65:1051–1057.

136 Christensen O (1987). Mediation of cell volume regulation by Ca^{2+} influx through stretch activated channels. *Nature,* 330:66–68.

137 Kasai H and Augustine G (1990). Cytosolic Ca^{2+} gradients triggering unidirectional fluid secretion from exocrine pancreas. *Nature,* 348:735–738.

138 Foskett J and Spring K (1985). Involvement of calcium and cytoskeleton in gallbladder epithelial cell volume regulation. *Am J Physiol,* 248:C27–C36.

139 Foskett J and Melvin J (1989). Activation of salivary secretion: Coupling of cell volume and $[Ca^{2+}]_i$ in single cells. *Science,* 244:1582–1585.

140 Schwab A et al. (1999). Migration of transformed renal epithelial cells is regulated by K^+ channel modulation of actin cytoskeleton and cell volume. *Eur J Physiol,* 438:330–337.

141 Kizer N et al. (1999). Volume regulatory decrease in UMR-106.01 cells is mediated by specific alpha 1 subunits of L-type calcium channels. *Cell Biochem Biophys,* 31(1):65–79.

142 Light D et al. (1999). Extracellular ATP stimulates volume decrease in Necturus red blood cells. *Am J Physiol,* 277:C480–491.

143 Marunaka et al. (1999). Roles of Ca^{2+} and protein tyrosine kinase in insulin action on cell volume via Na^+ and K^+ channels and $Na^+/K^+/2Cl^-$ cotransporter in fetal rat alveolar type II pneumocyte. *J Membr Biol,* 168(1):91–101.

144 Al-Habori M (1993). Mechanism of insulin action, role of ions and the cytoskeleton. *Int J Biochem,* 25(8):1087–1099.

Chapter Five

1   Blechschmidt E and Gasser R (1978). *Biokinetics and Biodynamics of Human Differentiation: Principles and Applications.* Springfield, IL: Charles C. Thomas Publisher, 285.

Postscript

1   In Booth ER (1905). *History of Osteopathy.* Cincinnati, OH: Press of Jennings and Graham, 63. [Work hereafter cited in text.]

Appendix

1   Still AT (1892). *The Philosophy and Mechanical Principles of Osteopathy.* Republished 1986. Kirksville, MO: Osteopathic Enterprise, 255. [Work hereafter cited in text.]

BIBLIOGRAPHY

I have included many important references here that support the thesis of this book. I have marked with an asterisk (*) those that were initially inspiring and fundamental to the process of my thinking and the development of this book.

BOOKS

By Andrew Taylor Still

*Still AT (1892). *The Philosophy and Mechanical Principles of Osteopathy*. Republished 1986. Kirksville, MO: Osteopathic Enterprise.

> This was Still's first book. He withdrew it from publication—even recalling distributed copies—almost immediately after it was marketed. Many of the passages in this book can be found verbatim in his subsequent books. However, references to biogen are found only in this book.

———— (1899). *The Philosophy of Osteopathy*. Fifth reprint 1977. Indianapolis, IN: The American Academy of Osteopathy.

> This is a smaller but no less valuable writing from Dr. Still.

*———— (1908). *Autobiography of Andrew T Still*. Reprinted 1981. Indianapolis, IN: The American Academy of Osteopathy.

> This is a colorful account of Still's life and times. We can gain many insights into Still's thinking from this autobiography, in which he describes his childhood, his struggles against the pro-slavery forces from Missouri, his battles in the Civil War, his questioning of the use of drugs, and his grief from the death of his children that stimulated his search for a better way. Accounts of his visions and dreams are included.

———————— (1910). *Osteopathy: Research and Practice*. Reprinted 1992. Seattle, WA: Eastland Press.

> This was Still's last book. It has a more philosophical tone and shows his obvious intent to relate the important aspects of his philosophy. For the first time in any of his writings, he gives instruction on technique.

About Andrew Taylor Still

*Booth ER (1905). *History of Osteopathy*. Cincinnati, OH: Press of Jennings and Graham.

> One of Still's early students and great supporters, Booth wrote this biography of Still and history of Osteopathy. It is very revealing about A. T. Still and the early years of the profession. It is out of print, but may be found online.

*Hildreth AG (1938). *The Lengthening Shadow of Dr. Andrew Taylor Still*. Kirksville, MO: Journal Printing Co.

> Hildreth was a student in Still's first class and one of Still's most devoted admirers, becoming the dean of the American School of Osteopathy and a lobbyist for the profession, achieving the legal acceptance of Osteopathy in several states. The book is out of print, but a few copies are available in the A. T. Still Osteopathic Museum in Kirksville.

Still CE, Jr. (1991). *Frontier Doctor—Medical Pioneer: The Life and Times of A. T. Still and His Family*. Kirksville, MO: Thomas Jefferson University Press.

> Still's grandson wrote this biographical account of A. T. Still in the context of the Still family.

Trowbridge C (1991). *Andrew Taylor Still: 1828–1917*. Kirksville, MO: Thomas Jefferson University Press.

> This is another excellent biography of A. T. Still. Carol Trowbridge researched local and long-distance sources for her information about Still. She speculates about his motivations and intentions.

Walter G (1992). *The First School of Osteopathic Medicine*. Kirksville, MO: Thomas Jefferson University Press.

> The long-time librarian at the Kirksville College of Osteopathic Medicine researched even outside the walls of the library to write this in-depth look at the early days at the American School of Osteopathy and beyond.

By William Garner Sutherland

Sutherland W (1990). *Teachings in the Science of Osteopathy*. Wales A (ed.). Fort Worth, TX: Sutherland Cranial Teaching Foundation.

This is a text on cranial osteopathy assembled from the writings and speeches of William Garner Sutherland, DO, by Anne Wales, DO, one of Sutherland's early students and dedicated assistants. Sutherland assured his students that his teachings were from the philosophy of Still who had taught Sutherland. Nevertheless, Sutherland's work and teaching expanded Still's philosophy because of Sutherland's discovery of the primary respiratory mechanism. This book reads easily and is less technical than other texts on the subject. It is a good resource about the cranial concept.

*——————— (1998). *Contributions of Thought.* Second Ed. Fort Worth, TX: Sutherland Cranial Teaching Foundation.

This is the original volume of collected writings of William Garner Sutherland, DO, compiled by his wife Adah Strand Sutherland and Anne Wales, DO. It reveals Sutherland's thoughts and philosophy.

About William Garner Sutherland

Magoun HI (1976). *Osteopathy in the Cranial Field.* Third Ed. Indianapolis, IN: The Cranial Academy.

This is a rigorous text on the topic of cranial osteopathy and is the ultimate resource for technical questions about the cranial concept.

*Sutherland A (1962). *With Thinking Fingers.* Indianapolis, IN: The Cranial Academy.

This is the delightful story of the professional development of Dr. Sutherland, as told lovingly by his wife, Adah.

By Other Authors

*Barral JP (1989). *Visceral Manipulation.* Seattle, WA: Eastland Press.

Jean-Pierre Barral has opened a new view of the body with visceral manipulation.

*Becker R (1990). *Cross Currents: The Perils of Electropollution; The Promise of Electromedicine.* Los Angeles: Jeremy P. Tarcher.

This book takes a deep look at the body's electrical system and how it is influenced by electrical pollution and medicine.

*Blechschmidt E (1978). *Biokinetics and Biodynamics of Human Differentiation.* Springfield, IL: Charles C Thomas.

This is a thorough explanation of mechanical and electrical forces within and outside the embryo and the major extra-genetic influences they have in its development.

*Capra F (1991). *The Tao of Physics*. Boston: Shambala.

Fritjof Capra reveals the similarities between the ancient view of mystics and the modern view of quantum physicists.

Dossey L (1999). *Reinventing Medicine*. New York: HarperSanFrancisco.

This book predicts the direction in which modern medicine will move, progressing from mind-body medicine to a new era of healing.

*Fulford R (2003). *Are We on the Path?* Cisler T (ed.). Indianapolis, IN: The Cranial Academy.

This is the collected works of Robert C. Fulford, DO. The view expressed by Fulford is a natural progression of the views of Still and Sutherland.

*Gabarel B and Roques M (1985). *Les Fasciae en medecine osteopathique*. Paris: Maloine.

Published in French, this book elucidates for the first time the details of a mechanism of the primary respiratory mechanism in the fascia.

Gerber R (1988). *Vibrational Medicine*. Santa Fe, NM: Bear & Co.

This provides a review of all the major systems and philosophies of healing that are based in vibration.

Handoll N (2000). *The Anatomy of Potency*. Hereford, England: Osteopathic Supplies.

This is an explanation of cranial osteopathy through modern physics by a British osteopath.

Hawkins D (1995). *Power vs. Force: The Hidden Determinants of Human Behavior*. Carlsbad, CA: Hay House.

This is a deep look at the spiritual determinants of the human condition and an exposition of the benefits of applied kinesiology.

McTaggart L (2002). *The Field*. New York: HarperCollins.

Written by a journalist who interviewed many top scientists in the realm of modern physics, this book explains the underlying field of All-That-Is.

*Nordenström B (1983). *Biologically Closed Electric Circuits*. Stockholm: Nordic Medical Publications.

Nordenström describes his experiments revealing circuits of electricity in the body. The potential in the tissues oscillates, according to his findings.

O'Connor J and Bensky D, eds. (1981). *Acupuncture: A Comprehensive Text*. Seattle, WA: Eastland Press.

O'Connor and Bensky translated this book from the original by the Shanghai

College of Traditional Medicine. It is a complete textbook, even dealing with questions that most non-Chinese ask about acupuncture. A good reference.

*Oschman J (2000). *Energy Medicine: The Scientific Basis.* Edinburgh, UK: Churchill Livingstone.

James Oschman uses scientific information to explain how healing happens. This is the most authoritative book on the subject of healing yet to appear in print. It includes a foreword by Candace Pert.

*Pischinger A (1991). *Matrix and Matrix Regulation: Basis for a Holistic Theory of Medicine.* Heine H (ed.) Brussels, Belgium: Haug International.

This is a very innovative and revealing book about the importance of the connective tissues in the function of the organism.

Pollack G (2001). *Cells, Gels, and the Engines of Life.* Seattle, WA: Ebner and Sons.

Pollack has succeeded in making it easy to understand the functioning of cells that exist in a gel state. In the process, he contravenes many popular assumptions about cell biology.

Rael J (2002). *In the House of Shattering Light: The Life and Teachings of a Native American Mystic.* Self-published.

We get a glimpse of the Native American mind in this eye-opening book by a Picuris-Ute mixed-blood medicine man who has also lived with and come to understand white Americans.

*Schwenk T (1996). *Sensitive Chaos.* Second Ed. London: Rudolf Steiner Press.

This is an artful exposition of the influence of the flow of water in the creation of forms in our environment and our bodies.

*Sheldrake R (1981). *A New Science of Life.* Los Angeles: Jeremy Tarcher.

Rupert Sheldrake proposes that all living things display their physical form because of a preexisting, unseen pattern of energy.

*Swedenborg E (1769). *Intercourse of the Soul and the Body.* Republished 1947. London: The Swedenborg Society.

This very small treatise from the mystic, physician, and scientist briefly summarizes his philosophy of creation and the relationship of spirit and matter. His other works are voluminous, detailed scientific books.

*Tiller W (1997). *Science and Human Transformation: Subtle Energies, Intentionality, and Consciousness.* Walnut Creek, CA: Pavior Publishing.

This is a startling exposition of the nature of matter and its relationship to health and healing.

*Tiller W, Dibble W, and Kohane M (2001). *Conscious Acts of Creation : The Emergence of a New Physics*. Walnut Creek, CA: Pavior Publishing.

> The phenomenal effects of intention are scientifically demonstrated.

Wilber K, ed. (1982). *The Holographic Paradigm and Other Paradoxes*. Boulder, CO and London: Shambhala.

> Prominent scientists and thinkers present in lay language many investigative currents that lead to a holographic paradigm.

JOURNAL ARTICLES

*Al-Habori M (1993). Mechanism of insulin action, role of ions and the cytoskeleton. *Int J Biochem,* 25(8):1087–1099.

> This investigator shows how ion concentration and cytoskeletal organization affects the activity of insulin on the cell.

Berridge MJ and Rapp PE (1979). A comparative survey of the function, mechanism and control of cellular oscillators. *J Exp Biol,* 81:217–279.

> This contains a complete list of the multiple oscillating mechanisms in the cell.

Christensen O (1987). Mediation of cell volume regulation by Ca^{2+} influx through stretch activated channels. *Nature,* 330:66–68.

> This is a review of the effects of calcium ion influx across the cell membrane on regulation of cell volume.

Clegg J (1992). Cellular infrastructure and metabolic organization. *Curr Topics Cell Reg,* 33:3–14.

> This classic article shows the relationship of the organization of the interior of the cell to metabolism.

*Deshmukh V (1991). Cascading morphoregulatory energy and the biological form: Theory and reality. *Med Hypoth,* 35:59–67.

> Using mathematics and cellular physiology, Deshmukh shows how the flow of fluid creates form in the organism.

Heisey S and Adams T (1993). Role of cranial bone mobility in cranial compliance. *Neurosurgery,* 33(5):869–876.

> This landmark paper disproves the Monro-Kellie doctrine. These authors state that the head is compliant, downgrading the doctrine to a hypothesis.

*Ingber D (1998). The architecture of life. *Sci Am,* 1998 (Jan.): 48–57.

This is a review article about tensegrity in the cell.

Jenkins CO *et al.* (1971). Modulation resembling Traube-Hering waves recorded in the human brain. *Europ Neurol,* 5:1–6.

This discusses the observation of motion in the brain that can be interpreted as the primary respiratory mechanism.

King H (1999). Articular mobility of the cranial bones: A review of the research and status of the support for further research on osteopathy in the cranial field. *Cranial Letter,* 52(4):11–13.

King recounts the evidence in the medical and scientific literature that supports the mobility of the cranium.

Levin S (1997). A different approach to the mechanics of the human pelvis: Tensegrity. In Vleeming A, Mooney V, Snijders C, Dorman T, Stoeckart R (eds.) *Movement, stability, and low back pain, The essential role of the pelvis.* London: Churchill Livingstone, 157–167.

This is a good description of the role of tensegrity in the function of the sacrum.

Michael D and Retzlaff E (1975). A preliminary study of cranial bone movement in the squirrel monkey. *J Am Osteopath Assoc,* 74:866–869.

This paper describes the motion of the skull bones of the squirrel monkey.

Moskalenko Y (2003). Wave phenomena; circulatory dynamics. Lecture given at PRM Research Symposium/SCTF Continuing Studies Program. Bloomingdale, IL. Publication pending.

Using transcranial dopplerography and plethysmography, Moskalenko shows the relationships of cerebrospinal fluid and blood flow to the movement of the skull bones.

Moskalenko Y *et al.* (1999). Periodic mobility of cranial bones in humans. *Hum Physiol,* 25(1):51–58.

This is a good study demonstrating cranial bone motion in the human.

*Nelson K, Sergueef N, and Glonek T (2003). Wave phenomena: The Traube-Hering oscillation and the cranial rhythmic impulse. Lecture given at PRM Research Symposium/ SCTF Continuing Studies Program, Bloomingdale, IL. Publication pending.

This is a demonstration of a simple measurement technique used to obtain valuable research information about the Traube-Hering wave, which many agree is synonymous with the primary respiratory mechanism. These investigators show that cranial manipulation affects the Traube-Hering wave.

*Pienta K and Coffey D (1991). Cellular harmonic information transfer through a tissue tensegrity-matrix system. *Med Hypoth,* 34:88–95.

This landmark paper demonstrates how vibrational information moves through the extracellular matrix into the cell.

*Vern B *et al.* (1988). Low-frequency oscillations of cortical oxidative metabolism in waking and sleep. *J Cereb Blood Flow Met,* 8:215–226.

These investigators demonstrate an oscillation of the concentration of metabolic factors in the cerebral cortex.

Wang N, Butler J, and Ingber D (1993). Mechanotransduction across the cell surface and through the cytoskeleton. *Science,* 260:1124–1127.

Research is reported showing that mechanical energy passing across the cell membrane induces chemical events inside the cell.

ABOUT THE AUTHOR

Robert Paul Lee, DO, grew up and went to college in the same locale in the United States where Andrew Taylor Still, MD, DO, experienced his revelations that led to his developing osteopathic medicine. Years before Lee became aware of the existence of either Still or osteopathic medicine, he would sit on the edge of "Mount Oread" at the University of Kansas gazing east into the broad valley where Still had read medicine under the tutelage of his father on the Wakarusa Shawnee Indian Mission. As an undergraduate, Lee majored in biochemistry and physiology. He went on to the Kansas City College of Osteopathic Medicine and completed his rotating internship at Doctor's Hospital in Columbus, Ohio. Later, he became determined to learn more about osteopathic medicine's treatment of health problems related to structure-function and completed a residency in Osteopathic Manipulative Medicine at the Kirksville College of Osteopathic Medicine. Lee then settled in Portland, Oregon, to work in the Department of Osteopathic Services at Eastmoreland Hospital, where he eventually became the director. He is currently in practice in Durango, Colorado. Lee has also trained under the auspices of the American Academy of Medical Acupuncture. He is active in the American Academy of Osteopathy, having served on the Board of Governors, the Louisa Burns Osteopathic Research Committee, and the Publications Committee. He also has served on the Board of Directors of the Cranial Academy and the Cranial Academy Foundation. Lee earned a Certificate of Competency from the Cranial Academy and a fellowship from the American Academy of Osteopathy. He is certified by the American Osteopathic Board of Special Proficiency in Osteopathic Manipulative Medicine and by the American Board of Medical Acupuncture.

INDEX

V

van der Waals forces, 209, 214
Vern, B., 199, 200, 246
vertigo, 141
Virchow, Rudolf, 72, 213
viscero-somatic reflex, 24-25, 27
viscero-visceral reflex, 24-25
vitalism. *See* life force/vitalism

W

Wang, N., 242
water, 260
    as body fluid, 171, 172, 188, 209
    in cells, 213, 246-47, 259, 261
    consciousness and matter, 106-11,
        185-86, 258
    distribution of, 179-80
    in ECM, 215, 216-18, 223-24, 228,
        229
    electrochemistry and, 171, 175-76,
        181, 208, 231
    hydraulic forces, 175
    hydrogen ion flow, 208, 209
    as information carrier, 187-88, 189,
        191, 215, 224
    life force and, 171, 172, 192
    light and potency, 188, 262
    metabolism and, 184, 185-87, 192,
        202, 263-64
    oscillations, calcium, 234
    oscillations, rhythmicity of, 191-201
    properties of, 175-81, 185-86,
        187-88
    proteins and, 179
    as spirit/matter interface, 174,
        188-90, 192, 237
Weaver, Charlotte, 6, 146-47
Wheatley, D., 248-49
Wilkinson Microwave Anisotropy Probe
    (WMAP), 96-97
Wiseman, N., 65

www.ingramcontent.com/pod-product-compliance
Lightning Source LLC
Chambersburg PA
CBHW052009030426
42334CB00029BA/3148